The End of Fear Itself

by

Steve Bivans

2016

First Edition

To Patience, for walking through the Forest with me.

Table of Contents

Introduction__ 1

Can't See the Tree for the Forest__ 13

But Trees Are Natural!___29

In the Shade of the Tree__41

One Big-Assed Tree__61

You're a Lumberjack and You're Okay__127

Conclusion__205

ACKNOWLEDGMENTS

As with every book, or major project, there are too many people to thank and I'll probably forget someone. But thank you-s are essential and something I love to do, so here it goes.

Thank you to my beautiful companion in life, Patience Felt, who has always lived up to her name. I've put it to the test many times and she's still here. She was also the main editor for this book, as she was for *Be a Hobbit*. If there are any spelling or grammatical errors, they *is* my fault. If there are too many commas, still, then the fault is mine, again.

Thank you to my family, especially my daughter, Samantha, who is always an inspiration to me. Thanks to my step-son, Duke, whose courage inspired an entire chapter of this book. Thank you to my parents, Sam and Linda Bivans, for always being there for me and for all of us, and for the lessons you taught me. Thanks to Greg and Linda Felt, for being my parents-away-from-home and for your generosity and hospitality. Thanks to the entire Bivans clan and the Felt clan! I love you all!

Thanks to my inspirational coach, Bobby Kountz, who has helped to push, pull, and drag me through the painful process of writing this book. I probably would have written it without him, but it would have taken a hell of a long time, and might have been a far inferior work. Thanks to Justin Finkelstein for being the 'man in the street' pushing us all to think big and to 'throw things against the wall to see if they stick.' It was through a discussion with him, on Anchor, that the spark for this book was ignited. Thanks to Greg Dickson and Alida McDaniel for helping me with my toxic emotions around money.

Thanks to Brad Fergusson for interviewing me about the book. Thanks also, to Brett & Tristan at The Crucial Team for having me as a guest on their YouTube channel, twice! Thanks to Meredith Arthur for the discussions on anxiety, overthinking, and fear, and for her hospitality on Beautiful Voyager. Thanks to all my friends on Anchor, who chimed in on numerous *waves* to discuss multiple topics on fear. Thanks to all my friends, everywhere, who have always supported what I do. Especially thanks to my good friend, James Coplin, for *not* telling me that I'm crazy for writing about modern Hobbits, and trying to do something impossible like End Fear Itself. And, thank you to my English professor, Dr. Nicole Nolan-Sidhu, for kicking my ass and helping me to become a better writer.

A very special thanks to my very good friend and client, Amber Lynne, for sharing her amazing struggle with me, and the world. Keep and eye out. She's coming your way.

Another special thanks to Tammy Shockley, who read through the majority of this manuscript for all of my errors, and crossed through my, too, numerous, commas.

A big thank you to my official LAUNCH TEAM, for helping to promote this book. I could not have done it without them: Tim Bivans, Adam Blackler, Heidi Coplin, Geralyn Glasser, Helen McVey Khan, Mary Cheyne, Alex Wisnoski, Diane Warren Anderson, Mike Myles, Brett & Tristan at Crucial Team, Katie Swanson, Nilgun Tuna, Cameron Parkhurst, Sandi Dearin, Derek Markham, James Brannon, Trinity Kathleen Tyndall, Caleb Grote, Chris Palmore at GratitudeSpace, David Lenander, April Streich, Allan Niass, Liz Pearson, Sharon Fischlowitz, Tim Ebl, Mimi Emmanuel, Bhoopathi Rapolu, Brad Fergusson, Richard Edgar, Razz Purser, Heather Jerebek, Holly Schultz, Tiki Tischeleder, Josias Arcadia, Heather Jayne Blenkinsop, Maureen Hark, See Xiong, Jackie Kennedy, Sam Eaton, Maurice Ehrlich, Christine Shyne, Big Dave Daily (Smith), Sharon Lowder Stutts, Brianna Hiroshi, Katy Lowery, Gbenga Akinwole, Nate Snyder, Ellie Leonardsmith, Taylor Kendal, Aaron Reynolds. Alida McDaniel, Rebecca Liles Kolb, Greg Dickson, Jim Saunders, Linda Felt, Craig Johnson, Chris Genge, Michael Zeitgeist, Michael Prywes, Adrienne Hardison.

FOREWORD

On June 23, 2015, I woke up and literally could not get out of bed. I was paralyzed by Fear and anxiety. For three straight weeks my mind had raced through the night. I had convinced myself that that my most ludicrous Fears would come to fruition. On that summer Tuesday morning, I could go no further.

I called friends.

One told me to see a conventional Western doctor first thing in the morning. Another suggested an Eastern medicine doctor. I couldn't wait any longer; I needed to see somebody right away.

I saw the Western doctor first, who recommended that I take anti-anxiety medication. The downside was that it would basically turn me into a zombie for weeks, which would get in the way of everything that I needed to do.

The Eastern doctor gave me 14 paper bags full of herbs, with the instruction that I should take it twice a day for two weeks. I knew this was a better long-term solution but that the effects wouldn't be immediate. I needed relief immediately, so I resigned myself to take the anti-anxiety medication for one day.

I took the drug and started right in on the herbs.

If I'd possessed the book you are holding now, I would have handled the situation very differently.

I met Steve Bivans in February of 2016, as we were both experimenting with a new audio, social media app: Anchor. Since then, we have become good friends and co-creators.

One day I shared with the Anchor community how upset I was after dropping my daughter off at the school bus. She was worried that the other kids were going to make fun of her because of the shirt that she was wearing. There was nothing out of the ordinary about the shirt, but when we she gets an idea into her head, it's hard to get it out.

After dropping her at school, I recorded a two minute audio message on Anchor to share how helpless and alone I felt because I didn't know what to do to support my daughter. I was afraid that I might have given her the wrong advice and there was nothing I could do, during the day while she was at school, to protect her from her peers.

Within minutes, dozens of people from the Anchor community chimed in to offer me comfort and advice and a long conversation ensued. Steve joined that conversation. He advised that simply because I *feared* screwing it up, likely meant that I was probably doing okay.

I had been to therapy before, but this conversation had the same impact with far less effort.

When my daughter came home later that day, I asked her how her how her day had been. My Fear had been for naught. Not one person had mentioned the shirt, all day.

A few days later, Steve shared the story of Silly Miss Tilly, a balloon artist who brings joy to hundreds, and has experienced a past that would cripple most people. Her story, which had been featured on USA Today, floored me. The fact that she had spent many years without her father—who had been in prison—brought back my Fears about parenting.

During a subsequent discussion about Fear, Steve declared he would write a book on the biggest topic that he could tackle - FEAR. Since I had just met Steve, I thought the conversation was going to end there, as most conversations do. But Steve wasn't kidding. He leapt into action and put pen to paper.

He posted *waves* on Anchor, reaching out to others in the community to get ideas on how they viewed Fear, how they would tackle this topic. Not all of the discussions were heavy and dark. Steve also mixed in lighthearted topics, challenging people think about Fear a little differently.

When Steve reached out to ask me to write the foreword to the book. I asked myself: "What about this topic is interesting to me?" And, more importantly, "How might this book change *my* life?"

As I mentioned, I've been crippled by Fear in the past. I wish I'd had this book that summer morning in 2015. But, as Steve points out in the pages of this book, the past doesn't exist anymore. All we *have* is the present.

In this book, Steve does an amazing job of weaving in stories of Fear and courage, along with tips that you can use to immediately get relief. He also lays out ideas and strategies that you can use on an ongoing basis to free you from Fear in the long term.

What Steve puts forward here is no less than a ***moon shot*** approach to ending Fear on a global level, beginning within ourselves.

Will he be successful? I say, "Yes!"

Will there still be some Fear in the World? Probably.

However, we will never know until we try.

I appreciate Steve for taking on the topic of Fear for everyone on the planet. Let's be honest, we will not conquer Fear, worldwide, until everyone *personally* conquers Fear. The lessons in this book will give you a chance to do something bold. Don't settle for *ordinary*. Here is your chance to be *extra*ordinary.

If you aren't operating at your highest level, this book is absolutely for you.

It is absolutely for YOU, NOW.

You may question some of the ideas in the book. Pay attention to those things that seem hard to swallow. They are probably things you need to hear.

I honor each and every one of you for taking on your life in an extraordinary way. Have an amazing life and thank you for spending the time to read this book. I promise, you'll not emerge from the Forest of Fear the same as you went in.

Justin Finkelstein
I help people find their voice, now.

If someone asked you what your life's mission or purpose was, could you answer it?

No?

Then I invite you to go to www.stevebivans.com,
subscribe to my blog
and get your
FREE **Fear-Less Life Mission Worksheet**!
You can do this at any time, of course. Just log in with your email address, and I'll send you the password and link to the worksheet!
Boom! Done!
With a Life Mission and No Fear, you'll be un-stopable.

"The only thing we have to Fear, is Fear Itself."
—President Franklin Delano Roosevelt

Introduction

INTO THE FOREST

A woman followed a man into the forest.

The man was a wolf.

The wolf was angry.

Amber Lynne was a popular children's performer in St. Paul. On the outside she was brighter than the sun, a flaming fireball rocket of fun. She could twist colorful balloon flowers, dogs, cats, aliens, laser blasters, you name it. She drummed, she danced, she sang. Everywhere she went, she brought smiles and laughter. She was the positive Pied Piper of the West Side.

When she landed on the West Side Farmers Market on Saturday mornings she transformed the space in an instant. As Silly Miss Tilly, in her electrified outfit—with iconic pink hair—she was instantly recognizable. Children erupted with glee. They ran to her, hugged her, sometimes tackled her to the ground. The next hour or so was always a blur of color: laughing children, popping balloons, beating drums, and dancing. The energy she brought to the space raced out at the speed and force of a tsunami, affecting everyone and everything in its path, transforming frowns, worries, Fears, and concerns into laughing hearts of joy.

Performing was Amber's oasis: a safe house where she could be herself.

While Amber worked in the Light, she lived in a Forest of Fear, with a wolf. The wolf was her husband and he was jealous of her sunshine. He lived only in the shadow of the Tree of Fear, deep in the dark Forest. The wolf was rarely amused, often angry, and always hungry. His name isn't important. We'll just call him Richard; no, on second thought let's call him Dick.

Dick was an abuser.

On the inside, Dick was a wolf and the wolf could appear at any moment. It required no moon, no magic spell to appear. Anything could trigger the transformation.

During a 4th of July family outing, the wolf was triggered by a common potion: an overabundance of alcohol and the opportunity to abuse something: a chicken. Dick turned his ire upon an innocent chicken, kicking it, presumably for his own amusement.

This *wolf-in-the-henhouse* attack brought condemnation from the owner and a well-deserved fist to the face. Man quickly turned to wolf and when Amber intervened, she became the focus of the his anger. The wolf stormed off into the Forest.

Amber raced in after him.

Moments after entering the Forest, Dick began to growl. Amber—shaking in Fear—turned to escape. The wolf pounced. His claws caught in her long, black hair, pulling as if to rip the scalp from her skull.

With open palms, he punched. He pushed her down into a dark, cold, shallow pool of water next to the forest path. She was submerged, gasping for breath every time she managed to push her head upwards out of the muddy pool.

"He's going to kill me!" raced through her mind, *"He's really going to kill me this time!"*

Then the wolf bit her.

Dick's teeth sank into her back. While pulling her hair with one fist, he drove his open palm down into her face with the other. Over and over and over again, howling obscenities, echoing off into the trees, "Fuckin' cunt! Stupid bitch!" He was out of control and the blood was in his eyes.

"Oh my God, Oh my God, Oh my God!!" she thought, each time she came up for air, the water, the mud, the rotting leaves clinging to her face, *"I'm not going to make it out of here!"*

Struggling to get free, to catch her breath, she pushed her body back against the wolf.

Suddenly his arms were around her throat. The wolf rolled her over. Now both victim and wolf were staring into the trees, while she desperately struggled to breathe. She was now lying on top of him, nearly blacking out from lack of oxygen and from the sheer terror that she might not live to see another day.

"This is it." the thought raced through her mind as the trees overhead became blurry, all things fading to white,

"This is it. I'm going to die."

No smiles.

No laughter.

No balloons.

No sunshine.

No happy children on a market morning.

Only silence in a darkening sky,

Only Fear, the howling of the wolf, and the faint outline of a Tree.

WHY YOU WANT TO FOLLOW ME INTO THE FOREST

"The entrance to the path was like a sort of arch leading in to a gloomy tunnel made by two great trees that leant together, too old and strangled with ivy to bear more than a few blackened leaves. The path itself was narrow and wound in and out among the trunks. Soon the light at the gate was like a little bright hole far behind, and the quiet was so deep that their feet seemed to thump along while all the trees leaned over them and listened. —J.R.R. Tolkien, *The Hobbit*

A little blonde girl wanders into the forest.

A girl in a red scarf carries a basket into the woods.

A boy and a girl are abandoned in the trees.

Another girl in a blue dress and ruby slippers, with her dog, drop from a storm-cloud and begin a journey down a yellow brick road through a forest full of lions, tigers, and bears.

Most of us know how these stories end.

Goldilocks encounters three bears, and barely escapes. Little Red Riding Hood was eaten by a wolf while delivering cake and tea to her ailing grandmother, only to be saved by a huntsman. Hansel and Gretel barely escape being eaten by an evil witch. Dorothy and Toto meet a Tin Man, a Scarecrow, and a Cowardly Lion while being pursued by the Wicked Witch of the West.

There is one central theme to all of these stories: Fear. Fear Itself.

These fairy stories are indicators of an ancient war against Nature—Mother Nature and *our* nature—that is still raging today. The Fear of Nature, of our possible annihilation, has driven us to the brink of realizing the very thing we fear. If we do not cease this war, we will lose it, and destroy ourselves along with millions of other species. In the meantime, and maybe even more important to us, the same Fears that drive us to destroy Nature, are destroying our individual lives.

Why Am I Writing a Book About Fear?

There are several reasons:

- Some are personal:
    - Because I struggle with achieving success
    - with staying focused
    - with distractions
    - with brain-spin and overthinking
    - with Fears abundant.
- Because I know I'm not alone in those Fears.
- Because I know the world can be a better place.
- Because I know Fear is preventing us from creating the world we *could* have.
- Because we can't fix the *world*; we can only fix ourselves: one individual at a time, looking *inward,* not outward.
- Because I genuinely want to help people to live a life of freedom, not of Fear.

What Is this Book Really About?

This book is about *why* we need to, and *how* we *can*, end Fear Itself. Fear Itself is the only real problem we face, but we can conquer it, if we are willing to do the work.

Is this Book for You?

No one is immune to Fear. And this book is for anyone who has ever suffered from Fear, which is everyone living on this planet. If you were immune, you wouldn't have begun reading this book.

I offer this book to those who are struggling in some area of their life: be that work, business, money, relationships, health, you name it. At the root of that struggle is a Fear, most likely several. Every block to your success in life is based on Fear. Don't believe me? Keep reading.

What Will You Discover?

- You'll discover the 5 Myths about the World's problems, and Fear Itself.

- You will discover the root of all of *your* problems, and the world's problems.

- You'll get a handful of proven methods to root out and remove those problems and any that you encounter in the future.

Who Am I to Write Such a Book?

That's an excellent question, and one that I've asked myself many times in the last eight months or so.

To answer it, I'll reveal one of my inner most Fears.

Quite frankly, I fear that I am inadequate and unqualified to write this book.

I'm not a professional psychologist or psychiatrist. I'm not a sociologist.

What I *do* have is years of experience analyzing people's lives, first as a friend, then as a personal coach and strategic advisor. Much of what I do is informed by years of training in the history and art of war. I've spent the last eight to ten years examining it in detail as a graduate student in history, and decades longer as an amateur. And is there anything humans do that is more filled with Fear than war? Probably not.

Even if I were *not* an historian of war, or an academic of any kind, I would still be fully capable of analyzing and writing about Fear. Who in this world is immune to its effects? No one.

Anyone could write a book on Fear, with full authority to do so. *You* could certainly write a book on it. There are probably many children who could. But only *I* can write *this book*, because I'm the only one in the Universe with my particular perspective. That doesn't make it better or worse, just unique.

These days, I'd much rather study peace. But standing in the way of peace is Fear. In the way of abundance, Fear. In the way of happiness, Fear. In the way of Joy, Fear. As F.D.R. said, "The only thing we have to Fear, is Fear itself," and we should *stop* fearing

IT! It's time to face Fear Itself, and kick its ass. So, I will take whatever criticism comes.

I am writing this book *in spite* of my Fears, because I *do* have them, not because I have already banished them to some sort of oblivion.

Other than my studies, I have 50 years of life experience, which certainly qualifies me to write about Fear. If that's not enough, then I offer one more qualification: I wrote it! There are tens of thousands of psychologists in the world, maybe millions, but they haven't written this book. They've written lots of books, for sure, but none of them have zeroed in on Fear in quite the way we're going to do in this book. What they *have* written about are various methods to uncover and tackle some of the most insidious problems that we face.

Most of the methods you'll find in this book didn't originate with me. I am indebted to many other psychologists, coaches, and other authors who blazed trails through other forests of human issues. All of them have faced criticism and derision at some point in their careers, but they stuck it out and have provided some useful tools to help bring down the Tree of Fear.

My goal is to bring them all together in one place to help you chop down your Tree of Fear and become the liberated, successful, happy person you were meant to be. Is that ambitious enough?

I am not a Zen Master of Fear. I still have Fears. There is an assumption of which I'm guilty: if someone is an author, they have the authority to write on a topic. While this may or may not be true, it doesn't mean they have all the answers, or that they have already mastered the problem and eliminated it from their own lives. They just had the courage to write about it.

I certainly have not mastered all of my Fears. I still have some. One of the main reasons I wrote this book was a selfish one; I wanted to figure out how to overcome my own Fears. So, while I may have given the topic more thought than some people have, I am very much on the journey *with* you. I might be the guide, but it doesn't mean I've already been there. But if you'll trust me, just a little, I think I can get us through the Forest of Fear to a different place: a Fearless peaceful world.

Imagine Your World Without Fear

What would such a world look like?

What would it feel like?

Imagine being able to experience *true* freedom. There is no freedom if Fear exists in your mind. It is the darkest of forests. Without Fear you are free to do whatever you want. You are powerful beyond anything you can currently imagine. You are in control of your own life: your business, your job, your relationships, your well-being, your health, your happiness, your peace of mind, and your future legacy.

Picture it.

How powerful would you be?

Would you be able, now, to change the world? Absolutely.

And what if thousands, millions, or billions of other people did the same? Would we even be human anymore? Or would we transcend our current state and evolve into something more than human?

Imagine a world without war, without violence of any kind, without intolerance and racism, without poverty, without greed, without corruption, without environmental destruction.

Is this even possible?

You're damned right it is. To believe otherwise is to accept that problems *created* by humans, can't also be *un*created by humans. It's an illogical assumption, and it's bullshit.

So let's get to work on it. Let's begin by looking at the 5 Major Myths about what's wrong with the world.

THE FOREST: FIVE MYTHS ABOUT THE WORLD'S PROBLEMS

The reason why humans haven't been able to solve the world's plethora of problems is due to 5 key myths or misunderstandings about what's wrong, and our ability to do anything about it. As we move through the book, we will address those myths and misunderstandings, simplifying what seems to be complex, and bringing the *impossible* into the realm of the *possible*.

Here are the 5 key myths:

1. **There are too many problems and they are too complicated to solve.**
2. **Fear is just human nature.**
3. **Fear is a good thing.**
4. **There are too many Fears; we'll never sort them out.**
5. **No one person has the power to change the world.**

LET'S GET GOING

Now is the time to end Fear Itself. It is up to you to do this for your own well-being. To stop at this point, would be a tragedy. On the other side of Fear is an amazing land of peace and freedom.

A word to the reader

If you stop here, there are two possible reasons:

1. You think my writing is crap and don't want to read any further.
2. You are *afraid* to read this book: This could be for many reasons. If this is the case, you need to read it more than anyone else, so read on!

Do the Work

This book is useless if you never implement the methods I've collected for you. So many people fail to implement the advice when they read self-help books. Then they wonder why the advice doesn't work; of course it doesn't work, if you don't *do it*.

So don't make that mistake. Read the book, pick a Fear to tackle, and start somewhere. It doesn't even matter where you start. Just start.

Let's get going. It's time to begin our journey into the woods, in our search for the Tree of Fear Itself. Grab your lunch, put on your riding hood, and let's head into the Forest with all the courage we can muster.

1

Can't See the Tree for the Forest

ARE THE PROBLEMS TOO MANY? TOO COMPLICATED?

"Fear is the original sin. Almost all of the evil in the world has its origin in the fact that some one is afraid of something. It is a cold slimy serpent coiling about you. It is horrible to live with fear; and it is of all things degrading." —L.M. Montgomery, author and poet

Probably the most common myth about our ability, or lack thereof, to solve the world's biggest problems is that there are just too many of them. Which one do we tackle first? Do we try to solve them all at once? Do we have the resources to do that?

Mostly, it seems, we have been attempting to solve them all at once, and we have failed miserably on all fronts. That's not to say that no progress has ever been made on some of these issues, but they are all still here. Whatever progress has been made is small in comparison to the magnitude of the problems.

A laundry list of those problems would include violence and war, poverty, greed, political corruption, racism, sexism, religious intolerance, nationalism, mental illness, failed healthcare systems, and environmental destruction of all kinds. We could list them till the cows come home, till our pens run out of ink, or my fingers drop off from typing this paragraph, and still not list them all. The problems seem infinite.

But is that true?

It certainly seems to be the case. I thought the same thing when I began the process of researching and writing *Be a Hobbit, Save the Earth*, a few years ago.

What if all of those problems were really just symptoms of one core problem: a root problem?

There is only ONE real problem in human affairs, and that is Fear. **Fear** is the root of *all* human-driven problems. Everything else is a *symptom* of Fear. That's not to say that the symptoms haven't become problems in and of themselves. If you have the flu virus (the root problem), the runny nose, the chills, the fever, the shakes, and the nausea might be symptoms, but they are also problems when it comes to functioning normally.

It is the symptoms that we experience directly and are often the things that we focus our attention upon. But it's a very bad doctor who contents herself with only treating symptoms. In the case of the flu it might be a deadly decision. In the case of our global problems, the result might be deadly, too, just on a massive scale that would make a flu outbreak look like a picnic.

We've been attacking symptoms for a very long time. To continue to do the same thing expecting different results is the definition of insanity, even if Einstein never really said it. It's true nonetheless. Maybe it's time to try something different? Maybe it's time to focus on the cause? Hell, what do we have to lose at this point?

Trapped in the Forest of Fear

Trapped in the Forest of Fear

Amber Lynne escaped death that day in the woods, but just barely. And only due to her love for her son, and for her calling: Smiles and Laughter. She managed to break free of the claws of her husband the wolf. But her escape was only temporary.

While charges were filed, she retracted them. In a scenario all too familiar in cases of domestic spousal abuse, he begged forgiveness and she gave it to him. Over and over again, he begged for forgiveness. But Dick had no intention of facing his inner wolf. He chose to ignore it, assuming he could control it on his own. He could not. Time and again the wolf returned. Time and again, Amber forgave him.

Why?

Why would such an amazing woman ever *be* with a wolf in the first place? And why would she *ever* allow him to return, again and again?

Fear is why.

And that's how Fear works.

In cases of abuse, the Tree of Fear becomes a Forest of Fears. Every Fear you can imagine grows in that dark Forest. The world outside is feared *more* than the world within. Once inside the Forest of Fear, it is nearly impossible to imagine that the outside world is any different, and more often than not, it looks even scarier. *The Devil we know* always seems preferable to the devils that *may be*. It is a Fear of the Unknown.

And that isn't the only Fear that imprisons one in the Forest. There are the Fears of Failure, of Criticim, of Being Wrong, of Loss of Status, of Not Being Good Enough, and a host of others that block the paths out of that evil wood. They are tangled roots that reach out to trip up the would-be escapee, briars that snag dresses and trousers of those who would try to run away. Escaping is a very difficult and dangerous endeavor.

Many never escape. They are consumed by the wolf, entirely. Many die in the darkness of their own, psychological Forest. Some, after decades of terror, die of so-called 'natural' causes, as if years of abuse have no 'un-natural' effects on one's health. We know it does. Others are murdered outright by their wolfish husbands.

THE FEARS THAT BIND US

It is easy for some to turn the blame of abuse upon the abused. Especially since many of them blame themselves to begin with. Amber did. After so many beatings and beratings, she began to believe the lies told to her by her wolfish husband.

"I must be the problem!" she thought, *"What is wrong with me? I must not be a good enough wife. Maybe if I stay quiet and not antagonize him."*

Such thoughts are erroneous. Abuse is never the fault of the abused. But Fear instills such belief in the mind and it is very hard to shake. Most never manage it. But these kinds of Fears, these kinds of beliefs, aren't only the bane of the abused. They afflict us all to one degree or another.

We are all victims of Fear. At some point or other, we all live in the shadow of the Tree of Fear, and we all spend time in that dark Forest. We are all under the spell of our own Fears and they sap the life from us, from our families, from our friends, from our communities, and they radiate out into the world, like a dark tsunami, obliterating much that is good, leaving pain and suffering behind.

Fear is the one real problem on Earth. If we can, as individuals, tackle our own Fears, the result will radiate outward to the rest of the world, much like the effects of a butterfly flapping its wings. For we cannot bring about an end to *all* Fear, everywhere at once. That is truly beyond the power of any individual, or indeed any group of people, governments, or organizations. We cannot *legislate* an end to Fear. It has been tried, for millennia, and has failed.

It must either be eliminated in the hearts and minds of each of us, one by one, or surrendered to entirely. If we do not tackle this problem, if we do not bring about The End of Fear Itself, then we have no hope to alleviate the symptoms. For the rest of our problems are merely that: symptoms of Fear Itself.

But I believe it can be done.

We *can* bring about the End of Fear Itself.

It will not be easy. It is not a smooth road to walk, but we are walking it anyway. Winston Churchill once said, "If you're walking through hell, keep walking." Don't stop. Don't look around; just keep going. The only way to rid ourselves of Fear is to walk through the Forest, find that Tree and bring it down, then walk right through to the other side.

Let's Find that Poisoned Tree

There are hundreds, thousands, maybe millions of trees in the dark Forest of the world's problems. But in the center of that deep, dark wood is the Tree of Fear. Its roots are deep, and they stretch out under the earth, intwining with the roots of all the other trees, seeding them, feeding them a poisonous nectar. They serve to obscure the father of all evil trees: The Tree of Fear Itself.

In the case of some of these problems the link to Fear is fairly obvious, while in others, the roots leading back to the grandfather of the Forest are long and twisted. But I assure you that, if there is a problem that humans face, a problem *created* by humans, Fear is at the root. You just have to keep hacking your way through the underbrush and sometimes dig below the dirt. But the connection is always there. Always. Let's do a little trailblazing. Break out your machetes and shovels, and let's put our backs into it. Let's see if we can expose those connecting roots.

AN INVENTORY OF PROBLEM TREES

What are the world's greatest problems? What trees lurk in that dark Forest?

Violence and War

This one is easy, which is why I put it at the top. All war and all forms of violence are deeply rooted in Fear. ALL war and violence. Without Fear, there would be no war, or any kind of violence between people. Period. So, if you want to end war, and all violence, you must seek an end to Fear Itself.

There are many surface causes of war, and violence of every scale, but they all boil down to a Fear in the end. To illustrate this point, I sat down with a good friend of mine, Dr. Adam Blackler, a professor of history at Black Hills State University, via Skype, to get his take on the root causes of World War II.

He happily rattled off many of them: The First World War and the Versailles Treaty—which crippled Germany economically, giving rise to political instability and, ultimately, the NAZI Party, nationalism, racial constructs, a zero-sum economic philosophy, and several other factors.

As we discussed this, it became clear that Fear was the base of every one of these issues. Nationalism is an expression of *us* against *them*, our culture versus the culture of some *other*. Why does that matter? Because we define our own culture in terms not only of what it *is*, but what it is *not*, i.e., the culture of that *other* people, over there. We fear that if we don't define our culture, our political identity, then we will be overcome by some other group's culture and identity.

Closely linked to that are economic factors. If the Earth's resources are scarce—we'll discuss whether or not this is *true*, later—then we have to expand to take control of them. This is the zero-sum philosophy operating in late 19th and throughout the 20th, Century. Unfortunately, we're still operating according to this philosophical construct. It's based entirely on one particular type of Fear: the Fear of Scarcity, which is rooted in a Fear of Death, or

Annihilation. Fear was the root of World War II, if you really want to dig below the surface.

Even at the personal level, violence is rooted in Fear. If a husband drags his wife into the woods and strangles her to death, it is an expression of Fear, likely several different Fears all piled up on top of one another. He fears that she will leave him (Fear of Loss), that his family and friends will think he's a loser if she leaves him (Fear of Criticism, Failure, Loss of Status), and we could go on for some time listing more and more of them.

Poverty

Poverty is driven by a Fear of Scarcity, one of the Fears that drive us into war and violence. This is more complex than violence and war, but it comes down to the fact that we create our own reality; we attract it. Mostly, we do this subconsciously. This is not an argument to blame the poor for being poor. Some financially rich people are just as guilty of the Fear of Scarcity, which manifests itself in the form of Greed. Greed and Scarcity are just manifestations of Fear. Scarcity is an illusion, a very powerful one for sure, but an illusion just the same.

I've only recently come to the conclusion that most of what we see as scarce, really isn't. Yes, there are some resources on Earth that are becoming scarce because we, as a species, are burning them up, or using them up, or polluting them up at such a rate that they can't replenish themselves, (fresh water, clean air, energy resources, food systems, other species). But to say that they are scarce is to somewhat resign ourselves to a fate that says, "There's no other way to do things." It is to assume that the way we *have* been consuming is the way that we *will* consume, or that it's the *only way* to use the resources that we have, or that it's even a *good* way to do it.

There are myriad ways to use our basic resources more efficiently, sustainably, even regeneratively. Scholars like Buckminster Fuller, in the middle of the 20th Century, proposed many viable plans and suggestions on how to solve these problems. Technology has leapedfrogged several times since his death. Everything he dreamed of is now possible with the technology we already have. But most people remain ignorant of his ideas, or the innovative ideas of other scientists, economists, and philosophers with solutions to the world's economic issues. Our resources aren't really scarce; we're just wasting them.

Ignorance

This ignorance of new technologies and ideas isn't entirely the fault of the individual, though all of us are ultimately responsible for what we know or do not know. Even ignorance, especially the willful variety, is based in Fear. While it is perfectly natural to be ignorant of certain ideas or facts—we can't know everything there is to know—when we reject the truth or facts because they don't fit our version of the truth, we are practicing willful ignorance.

Why? Because we have a deep seated Fear of Being Wrong, (something we'll talk more about later.) The willful ignorance of people in power tends to drive overall ignorance amongst the rest of the population. If you have leaders who are afraid to be wrong, they will protect their sense of *rightness* by skewing the education of their people. This happens everywhere on Earth. Some of them can't really claim ignorance; they know quite well that there are solutions to many of these problems. Why do they do nothing? Simple. They're corrupt.

Politics and Corruption

All politics is rooted in Fear.

I know that's a bold statement, but I'll stand on it. Any form of governmental control, beyond a tribe choosing someone to organize the hunt, is based in Fear.

Think about it for a minute. Thousands of years ago, when villages, towns, and cities began to spring up in the Fertile Crescent, India, and China, the people chose leaders to write and enforce laws.

Why?

At first is was to organize the building of structures: temples and systems to water the crops. Large, time-limited projects need central organization. Even tribes had leaders. Most of the time it was a group of elders serving to organize things like hunting and gathering of food. Fear probably wasn't a major component of that, though there were probably times that prehistoric humans needed those same leaders to lead them into battle against their neighboring tribes. Conflict of this sort, as far as we can tell, has been with us for a very long time.

Once humans discovered agriculture and settled down into towns and cities, their collected wealth—usually food stores—became a sitting target for others. It's in this period that we see the rise of the *Big Man* of politics: lords and kings, and a new social group, the aristocracy. This is fully rooted in the Fears of the Other, and of Scarcity. And as soon as you have government of this nature, corruption follows like wolves follow little girls carrying baskets to grandma.

Governmental corruption is a massive topic these days, not that it was ever *not* a topic of discussion. It's an ancient tradition and one that is very difficult to fight. There's a lot of money injected into our political systems, worldwide, and money talks.

Corruption itself is based in Fear, too. It's very much based on the Fears of Scarcity and Loss of Control. The pursuit of power, for the sake of it, just like the pursuit of money simply to possess it, is corrosive: a mask for people who feel that they have no control in their lives. They have a Fear of the Loss of Control.

A Broken Healthcare System

Who would argue that the American system of health-care is functional? Not many. *Why* it's broken is hotly debated, but there are some central reasons. One is that our political system is so corrupt, and as a result, so is our economic system. The fact that the U.S. healthcare system—and the use of the word 'system' is grossly out of place—is so out of whack rests squarely on the fact that it has become a 'free-market' commodity, instead of a benefit for the tax-payer. You can get really great healthcare if you have a shitload of money. If you don't? Let me tell you, people; you are fucked. There's no soft way to put it.

I am well acquainted with just how bad it can be, even though I have 'insurance.' It covers nothing but 70 percent of major medical expenses, after a huge deductible. Essentially, the only way it's of use to me is if I have a heart-attack and end up in the emergency room or on the operating table. But even then, the 30 percent copay would destroy our financial situation and put us out of house and home.

I spent some time the other day discussing this *system* with one of my very good friends, Dr. Heidi Coplin, who's been working in it for nearly 20 years. Most of what she had to say, I'd heard before, especially since she and I and her husband have spent a great deal of time discussing it over cocktails. But the themes that came out of our talk all revolved around economic pressures from insurance companies and drug companies, and the corruption of our government by those same interests in the pursuit of more and more profits. Where does this drive for more and more come from? Greed, which is a product of the Fear of Scarcity.

Enabling that greed is the advertising/marketing arms of those corporations, and our commercial media culture that tells us every day, all day, that the solution to our health problems comes in pill form. "Just take this pill, and everything will be awesome!" But we all know, deep down, that it's just snake-oil and bullshit. We are addicted to instant cures, and instant everything.

And the real cure for most of our health issues? Real food.

Commoditized Calories, Not Nutrition

The world's food system is to blame for much of our health problems, along with the instant gratification culture we live in. Our over-paced lives, running around chasing dollars, seemingly for the sake of it, drives us to ignore one of the most important things, if not *the* most important things, we can do for our health: eating good food. And when I say *good*, I do not mean, that it just *tastes* good. That is important, very important as far as I'm concerned, but it also has to be *real* food, i.e., not injected with toxic chemicals, pumped full of corn sugar, salt, and lab-conjured false fats.

Food, like our health, has become a commodity to be sold to the highest bidder and traded like Boardwalk and Park Place.

What do you think drives this shift from nutrition to caloric commodities?

Fear drives it.

The same Fears that drive our entire economic

system: Fear of Scarcity and Poverty, and its product, greed. But there's also an underlying Fear that allows these corporations to yank us around by our emotional chain, and that is the Fear of Inadequacy: that we are simply not *good enough* if we don't buy their products.

Destruction of the Environment

Hand in hand with the corruption of our political, health, and food systems, comes the destruction of the natural world, via climate change, pollution, and the waste of the natural resources that we depend upon for our very survival. All of this is driven by the Fear of Scarcity.

While some natural resources *are* scarce, they are made so by our very Fears. By looking at the world as a place of scarcity, we scramble to extract as much of the abundance as we can, instead of focusing our energy upon finding ways to use the resources in a sustainable or regenerative way. The result is what we have: hunger, fresh water scarcity, pollution of our air, water, and earth. But this isn't the way it *has* to be, only the way we *think* it has to be.

Intolerance

All forms of intolerance — racism, sexism, religious and ethnic conflict — are based solely in Fear: the Fear of the Other, or the Unknown. There is no basis for intolerance other than Fear. This is one of the most destructive manifestations of Fear, and is also one of the major causes, if not *the* major cause, of much of the world's violence and war.

This Fear is an old one. While based partly on the Fear of Scarcity — the scarcity of resources — it's also rooted in the Fear of the Unknown, as well as the Known. If we meet another group of people, and we know nothing about them, then it is natural to be fearful until we have assessed whether or not they are truly a threat to us. Of course, no one *need* be a threat. Threats are *created*.

Most of the time, the intolerance and resulting violence spawns from a mutual Fear of the Unknown; both sides are ignorant, and therefore assume the worst. More times than not that assumption escalates to conflict, which leads both groups to create a Fear of the Known; both sides are now *known threats* to each other, and we're off to the races.

If we want to end intolerance of all kinds, then we have to put an End to Fear Itself. There has never been a law that has effectively ended intolerance. Laws may curb certain manifestations of it but laws are always *re*active; they are reactions to real or perceived problems. They do not *pre*empt the act they set out to curb, however much our lawyers and politicians might argue that they do. They might keep the 'honest' honest, sometimes. Mostly, they just give us a way to punish the transgressor, if and when we catch them stepping over the line. This does little for the victim of the crime.

Hate and Indifference

What are the roots of Hate?

I think it's the border between the Fear of the Unknown — the other that we don't know — and the Fear of the Known — the other that we *do* know and have past negative interactions with, or that we have been told we will have negative interactions with. We don't have to personally experience negativity from another person, or group of people, to consider them a threat; we can be educated to *think* that way, by our parents, our schools, and society at large. We can be *conditioned* to Fear the other.

And if there is any evidence whatsoever that that person or group have *ever* been a *real threat*, (i.e., one of them has been aggressive, or nasty, or just a pain in the ass,) then our suspicious minds create a stereotype around that event, to paint the person or group as a threat.

More often than not, this scenario applies to larger groups of people based on race, religion, or culture. But the roots of the problem stem from one-on-one experiences that each of us have with people from another group — as if groups actually existed. They don't, since they are constructs of the mind, not actualities. But perception is reality, as they say.

We have *created* these groupings in our minds, and so they exist, for us. The fact that we can *uncreate* them rarely occurs to us. They seem as if they are concrete. That person is *black*, or *hispanic*, or *Muslim*, or *white*. These are self-imposed boxes that we use to label other human beings, hell, to label our*selves*! I am white. But am I really? Mostly, I'm kind of beige, or tan, depending on what time of the year it is. It's all arbitrary bullshit. I could apply a hundred or a thousand labels to myself. But are any of them really helpful to understanding what makes Steve Bivans tick? Maybe, but only to a superficial degree.

And so, we have personal experiences, negative ones, with a person from another mentally constructed group and then, as we have more of them we begin to form our own picture of the group as a whole. We extrapolate the data to paint the entire group — something we (and they) created in the first place — with a broad brush as a group to be distrusted, disliked, or even hated.

This is the root, as I said, of racism, both on an individual and systemic level. It's what perpetuates it, even in an age when you would think such ridiculousness would have long been dead. Hate and intolerance is one of the driving reasons I decided to write this book in the first place. When our Fears reach the point of hate, violence is coming around the bend. And it does. It is the supreme expression of Fear: a Fruit of the Tree of Fear. It is the nastiest fruit that the tree produces, and it grows on the limb of intolerance.

The Opposite of Love?

It also grows on the limb of Indifference, which is really the opposite of love. Hate isn't the opposite of love. Hate requires us to actually focus on the person or persons that we hate. We have to think of them as at least somewhat human, as being like us in some small way.

But indifference allows us to relegate people, animals, the planet, to a category of inconsequential. This is the dangerous, slippery slope that leads to mass murder on the scale of the Holocaust. Most people think that hate is what drove the Nazi State to such extremes. I don't think so. I think hate was the road by which they reached it. The years of scapegoating Jews and others for the ills inflicted upon the Germans after World War I, certainly caused many a German to hate them. But after a while, the hate subsided and indifference set in. And then the trains began to move, and the smoke went up the chimney.

Eventually, the person you hate becomes non human, non existent. And that is a very nasty place to be. It leads to crimes of the most appalling nature. And some might argue that this is the *natural state* of humans: to be violent and intolerant: a persuasive myth, indeed.

GOODIE BASKET ONE: A SIMPLIFIED WORLD

At the end of each section, I'm going to give you a Goodie Basket, kind of like Red Riding Hood took to her Grandmother. It will be a short-list of the most important takeaways. That way, when you come back to the book later, you can look in your Goodie Baskets to remind you what you need to work on, or remember.

Your First Goodie Basket:

- There's only **ONE root problem** in the world: **Fear Itself.**
- All the other problems are *symptoms* **of Fear Itself.**

2

But Trees Are Natural!

THE MANCHINEEL: A 'NATURAL' TREE OF FEAR

"The oldest and strongest emotion of mankind is fear." —H.P. Lovecraft, author and one scary mutherfucker

When I began writing this book, I created a massive mind-map to try to make sense of such an enormous complex topic. I didn't have a huge blackboard on which to draw this map, and I wanted a permanent version of it to refer to, so I went out into my garage, grabbed one of those huge lawn-clipping bags you get from the hardware store. I took it back inside, got out some scissors and cut it open so that it laid out flat. The thing covered the entire kitchen table.

Then I got to work.

I spent hours scribbling terms on that paper with Sharpies. Then I drew lines connecting all of them, and eventually I came up with the key points or categories of Fear, or at least what I thought they were at the time. But it was still very confusing. What I needed was a metaphor, an illustration of how Fear grows, how all the categories flow into one another. I needed an image that everyone could relate to. That's when the idea of the Tree of Fear hit me.

I walked over to the small chalkboard we have in our kitchen (the one that was too small for the mind-map) and I began to draw a tree. The tree I drew was actually pretty good, surprisingly good given my lack of artistic ability. I then labeled the various parts of the tree with the categories of Fear as I then saw them.

I stood back.

I looked over my work.

I was pleased.

But then a thought ocurred to me, *"This is a really pretty tree. I love trees. Trees are awesome. Why would anyone relate a tree to Fear? That's ridiculous!"*

My next thought was that maybe there was a tree, somewhere in the world, that wasn't so pretty, or so nice, that would serve as a model for my Tree of Fear. And thanks to Google, I found it.

Introducing the Real-Life Tree of Fear

In the Caribbean, there's a tree that can kill you.

To eat its fruit brings painful suffering, sometimes death.

The natives use the sap of the bark to make poison darts for hunting.

The Manchineel Tree is a tree you want to avoid. It produces loads of small, green, apple-looking fruit, about the size of a large crabapple. But don't eat them! They're quite poisonous, and if ingesting the fruit doesn't kill you, you'll probably wish you were dead.

And it's not just the fruit that will kick your ass; the entire tree is toxic — roots, trunk, bark, branches, and leaves! Just *standing* under a Manchineel Tree can be a horrifying experience, especially if it's raining. Many seek shelter under the shady eaves of this tree, only to be drenched in drops of acidic sap dripping from the leaves when it rains and falls on the unsuspecting shade-lover. The result is severe rashes and blistering of the skin.

In the 15th and 16th centuries, Spanish explorers dubbed it the *arbol de la muerta*: the Tree of Death. Natives have long used this sap as a poison for their blow-darts and arrows, for hunting and fighting. In fact, Ponce de Leon suffered a wound from such an arrow in a battle with the Calusa tribe in southern Florida, and subsequently died from it.

Strangely enough, there's only one animal known to eat from this cursed tree: the Striped Iguana, a reptile. Lizard Brain food, anyone?

Fear is such a tree.

The Manchineel Tree might be toxic and sometimes kills its victims, but the Tree of Fear is deadly. It kills dreams and aspirations, destroys lives, loves, and minds, and if it doesn't kill you immediately, it can transform a life into a sort of *walking death*. Just like the Manchineel, the roots, branches, and trunk of the Tree of Fear carry a poisonous sap, as well.

While trees are quite natural, some of them can kill you. All of them can, if they fall on you. Fear is natural as well, but that doesn't mean we should stand under it, climb it, swing around in its branches or eat its fruits. Let's examine the true nature of Fear and determine if it necessarily has to be part of our own.

Can We Change Human Nature?

Is It Human Nature to Fear?

If Fear is the only real problem, how come no one else is calling for the end of it? Why isn't there already a massive movement to eradicate it, tons of books written about it?

To be fair, there *are* people calling for its demise, and there's a small movement out there with Fear in its sights. I think the reason it hasn't gained enough traction, to date, is because there is a persistent age-old myth that Fear is simply a natural part of existence, for animals and humans alike.

It's just Nature.

And it's human nature.

Fear is everywhere, so much so that our attention is drawn elsewhere. We do not focus on the mundane, the ordinary, the normal, and Fear is about as normal as it comes. It goes unnoticed, precisely because it is so prevalent and pervasive. Want to hide something? Do it in plain sight. Since Fear has been with us since the beginning, at least some forms of Fear, we have come to accept all forms of it as normal, as part of human nature. But is it? And if it is, does it have to be?

Can we change human nature?

What Is Human Nature?

Are humans just naturally fearful, violent, self-centered, and stupid?

This often seems to be the case when we look around at all the problems in the world. It was my central belief for a very long time. As a young man, I abandoned college in the first year and a half, then spent the next 18 years or so, struggling to survive in a world that did, indeed, seem overly complicated, evil, and violent. It seemed that the human race was doomed by its own, nasty, brutish, and short-minded nature.

This is an argument articulated by the 17th Century, political philosopher, Thomas Hobbes, who had the unenviable misfortune to live through the English Civil War, a particularly bloody war, as wars go. And it colored his view of human nature in a very negative light.

The term *human nature* gets a lot of play. We throw it around all the time, mostly to explain all the negative crap that we see other humans doing in the world.

But what is it?

What do we really mean when we say *human nature*?

Defining *human nature* is a very difficult thing to do, though many have tried, and many more are still attempting to do it. The more I look for this elusive thing, the less I find it. Beyond the natural drive to survive, there isn't much else that is 'natural' about humans, including Fear Itself.

For most of my life, I've was a fan of old Hobbes and his nasty, brutish, short philosophy.

Many still subscribe to this view of our basic nature.

Instinct vs Drive

For much of the 19th and early 20th Centuries, Western scientists, philosophers, and eventually psychologists, liked to refer to our basic natures as *instincts*, essentially our animalistic programming that led us to seek food, shelter, to procreate: basically, to *survive*. This is our basic *survival instinct*, that most of us still throw around in conversation.

But in the later 20th, and now into the 21st Century, the popular term has become *drives*. We are said to have *drives* to do all of those things we once had instincts towards. It's as if there is some little guy in our heads, our subconscious, behind a metaphorical steering wheel, driving us around like Miss Daisy from place to place, from the buffet table to the bedroom, and to the closet to get a coat so we don't freeze our ass off in a Minnesota Winter.

What the hell is all this? Who's driving?

Who is in control? Are we little more than robots, shuffling around after sex, controlled by some adolescent god, drooling on himself? Or are we just a bunch of fuckin' billiard balls on the Great Pool Table in the sky, knocked around by an invisible cue, wielded by the invisible hand of an invisible pool shark somewhere out around Ursa Minor?

Do we have free will, or not? Are we masters of our own destiny, or pawns in a great chess match in Heaven?

I would argue that, regardless of who is in charge—if anyone other than ourselves—we still have choices to make. At least that's the only truly sane way to approach life, and the one I will work from. But where does it leave us when it comes to Fear? Is it just part of our nature, unchangeable, untouchable?

I don't think so. In fact, I'm just going to say, NO, it is not a foregone conclusion in our lives, and yes, it can be changed.

Is it possible to End Fear?

This is a great question and I think it has at least two answers.

I don't think we can eradicate *all* Fear completely. Some forms of Fear are quite natural, as we'll discuss in depth. For instance, the Fear you feel when confronted with a large stranger in a dark alley at night in a rough part of town. That kind of Fear is a natural survival instinct, and as such, will never be eradicated. How we *respond* to such Fears is another story. Our response is always under our control.

What we *can* eradicate is Fear *Itself*, which is to say, Fear Incarnate, as a thing-a force-a living, breathing actor in our minds. *That* is what I am focusing on in this book. I believe, nay, *know* that this can be accomplished. I've seen it happen in other people, and I've managed to accomplish it in my own life, to a large extent. I'm still working on my own Fears, just in case you were thinking I was some kind of walking Buddha or something. I assure you, I am not. I have Fears, too.

What we are attempting to do in this book, is not to wave a magic wand and make all Fears disappear, worldwide. That isn't possible. What we *are* going to do, however, is to obliterate the *Thing*, called Fear.

FEAR AS A THING

In order to tackle a problem, we must first determine what that problem is. Part of that is to define the terms. The term I've chosen to use for our problem is Fear.

But what is Fear? How do we define it? This sounds like a simple enough question, but that's deceiving. It's not at all simple.

Fearing Fear Itself

During the research for this book, I had many discussions on the topic of Fear on a new, social media app, called Anchor. It's unique in that it is solely an audio format; all the posts are short audio recordings. It's pretty amazing actually.

I used the app to pose questions to the community about Fear, and in one of those discussions, my good friend Antonio Vereen, a veteran of the U.S. military, took umbrage with my use of the word *Fear*. For him, it is a very negative word, and emotion. He basically argued that he did not have Fear, but was instead, on occasion, *afraid*.

I'm sure his distinction stems from his training in the military. Fear is a real problem in all armies, throughout history. Fear can destroy a military unit and reduce it to a pile of bones and blood, if not checked quickly.

Nouns, Adjectives, Verbs: Fear Becomes an Actor

Antonio's distinction between Fear and being afraid is interesting. It's the difference between a noun and an adjective. When we 'noun' something, we give it form, and a certain reality, beyond just an emotion or idea. It becomes solid, in a way.

As a noun, Fear becomes a thing, but not an inanimate thing, like a table; it becomes an *actor* in our lives. It takes on the role of the subject in a transitive sentence—sorry for the grammar geeky stuff. In other words, Fear becomes personified, an actual force of action, an *actor* in the story we call Our Life. As a noun, we can refer *back* to Fear, in a sentence, "The only thing to fear is Fear *itself*." Since it has become a noun, we can use pronouns to refer to *it*.

Of course, we use pronouns to refer to inanimate objects, too. We can refer to a table, for instance, as *it*. But how often do we say, "The table *itself*?" Not very often. *Itself* is usually reserved for very special nouns, things we perceive as having a *self*, an inner being, or at least things that we want to put special emphasis upon.

Afraid: the Distance of Adjectives

Antonio's use of the word *afraid*, is interesting, because it's an adjective, instead of a noun.

An adjective is just a descriptor of a state of being, which is more transitory in nature than a noun. It's less solid, which may be the reason the military prefers the word *afraid* as opposed to Fear. It also puts a bit more distance between the Fear and the person feeling the Fear. It suggests that the person hasn't *identified* with their Fear but are in the process of *experiencing* it.

Fearing: the Transitive Nature of Fear

The only thing more transitory than an adjective is a verb, which depicts action or state of being. Instead of "I have a Fear," we could say, "I am fear*ing*," which means "Right now, I am in a state of Fear," not constantly carrying around a 'thing' called Fear.

In this state of mind, one can realize that *to fear* is a transitory thing, not a solid, negative object that is always in our minds and always there to block us. It isn't a little chauffeur in our brain, driving Miss Daisy around, in other words. It will dissipate over time, or it can. Fearing is only truly destructive when it becomes Fear: once it becomes a noun and decides to take up residence in our minds as a permanent force, as the driver.

Even as a verb, fearing can be destructive if it causes us to freeze when we should act. In a military unit, this is the kiss of death, and the reason why they adopt such mantras as *'fire and maneuver,'* because sitting still when under fire is not a good thing to do. Your enemy can zero in on your position and bring intense fire upon you. If you are in constant motion it is very difficult to do that. It's harder to hit a moving target than a stationary one. That's a very good lesson for life, as well.

There IS No Stationary

To remain stationary is an illusion anyway. Nothing in the entire Universe is stationary. Every rock on the Earth is moving through space at an alarming rate, because the Earth is moving through the Solar System, which is moving through the Milky Way, which is in turn racing through the Universe. Nothing is stationary. But when we think of ourselves as 'not moving,' we allow our minds to be controlled by negative thoughts, more often than not, instead of positive ones.

And if nothing is stationary, neither is Fear. All Fear is really fear*ing*. In reality, Fear doesn't exist. It is an illusion created in our minds. We give it solidity. We identify with it. It becomes a solid, negative Thing in our lives. But it isn't a given part of human nature. We can escape it. We *can* transform our own nature.

FROM HOMO SAPIENS TO HOMO LĬBĔR

What I'm calling for is nothing less than an evolutionary step. I'm challenging you, myself, and the entire Human Race, *Homo sapiens*, to consciously create our own evolution—which we now have the power to do—to become a new species. Yes, that's what I said.

The entire history of evolution has been an unconscious process of development, from single-celled organisms, crawling around in some muckity muck in the distant eons of time, to all the wonderful species of animals and plants that we have today.

And I'm *not* going to perpetuate the myth that humans are the most evolved species on the planet. That is simply arrogance, and it's led to the destruction of many other forms of life. We have no objective evidence, and certainly nothing constituting *proof*, that we are more intelligent or evolved than any other species. We are just different.

We don't know what broccoli thinks, for instance. Maybe all the broccoli on the planet think we're fuckin' stupid, uppity apes! We don't know. I'm certain that my two cats think precisely that. You can read it in their expressions and body language. I dare anyone to look my Squishy Kitty in the face and not feel inferior.

But whether we're inferior to kittens and broccoli, or not, I'm suggesting that it's time for humans to manifest their own evolution, consciously, into a new form of the *homo* genus, what I suggest should be called, *Homo lĭbĕr*: Liberated Mankind.

While Fear may be based in our past evolution as a species, and while we won't be able to end all forms of it, we can certainly end its hold on us. We can liberate ourselves from its destructive *power*, the chains that keep us down, that destroys our lives and the lives of billions of others. We can become something new: a species no longer yanked around by our Fears. What a world *that* would be!

Imagine it, for a minute. Let's put on our John Lennon tinted glasses, and imagine a world without Fear, a world without war, a world without poverty, a world without racism and intolerance. Can you? If you can, even for a moment, keep reading. I believe we can have such a world. I'll go even further in that belief. I believe we WILL HAVE IT! Yeah, I said it. Deal with it. Read on.

GOODIE BASKET TWO: NATURE OR NO?

- **To be *afraid*** or to be fear*ing* is natural.
- To have Fear Itself, a noun, might be natural but it **ain't helpful**.
- **We *can* change our nature** by eliminating Fear Itself, the destructive kind of Fear.
- We can **elevate our species** from *Homo sapiens to Homo Lĭbĕr*, from Fearful thinking mankind, to Liberated mankind.

3

In the Shade of the Tree

CAN FEAR BE A GIFT?

On a hot, summer day, the shade of the trees is a welcomed thing. Even the shade of the toxic Manchineel Tree might be helpful on a blistering day in the Caribbean. But don't stand under it for long, or you'll pay a painful price. Fear, like the Manchineel, might serve a purpose at times. But it's not a place to stay.

I've often argued that Fear serves a very good purpose.

Fear is good.

But is this true? I'm going to argue both sides of it, but essentially I'm going to suggest, very strongly, that Fear *Itself* is *never* a good thing. The distinction is in the *Itself* part. There is at least one form of Fear that can be very useful, in actual dangerous situations, or situations that we think *might* be dangerous. Most of us, however, are so distracted by senseless Fears that we don't even hear, or listen to, the tiny voice in our head that says, *"Hey, that dark shadow in the alley might be a mugger!"*

Fleet-Footed Fear

I heard footsteps behind me.

And then the whispering of voices: two voices.

There were at least two men following me down Queen Street, and they were gaining on me.

Fear crept up my spine, I quickened my pace.

In 1991, I was 25 and full of piss and anger. I had already lost at marriage and business, which is quite an 'accomplishment' for someone so young. I hated the world and most everyone in it. I had a shitty job as a burger flipper at Burger King, standing in grease all day in a polyester costume, serving up slop to people who obviously didn't care enough to eat decent food. And the pay was truly *awesome*: minimum wage, which means that if my asshole boss could have paid me less, he would have.

I worked 5 or 6 days a week usually, and when I wasn't at work shaking fries and assembling Whoppers, I was either walking *to* work, *from* work, or sitting on my futon in my roach-infested apartment listening to Pink Floyd—happy music there, my friend—

and drinking heavily: mostly the cheapest beer I could find or very cheap, blended whiskey, shit like Traveler's Club—five dollars a fifth: Hell Yeah. Good times, my friend.

One Friday afternoon, pay day, I took my winnings home on foot. No one was available to give me a lift home that day, so I hoofed it in my soleless shoes. When I say sole-less, I mean it. I had literally worn out the front half of my crappy tennis shoes on the bottom side. Most people didn't know this, of course; they couldn't see the bottoms. But I could feel them. I also didn't wear socks, so essentially, I walked barefoot everywhere I went. And the streets I walked on in New Bern, N.C. weren't paved with gold, I assure you. Mostly, they were paved with asphalt, concrete, dirt, and glass of the broken variety.

But glass didn't usually penetrate my feet those days; they were as hard as the pavement underneath them: hobbit-like feet. I was used to feeling the pavement, the dirt, and the glass.

Anyway, I left work that Friday and stopped by a bank on the way home, which was conveniently located right next to a liquor store. I popped in there a moment later and picked up a fifth of something: probably Traveller's, which is a really shitty whiskey blend. I don't recommend it. I wouldn't recommend much of anything I did, or drank, in that period of my life.

The cashier slid my bottle of poison into a brown paper bag and I was back on the sidewalk, strolling at a quick pace to get back to the roaches, my futon, and the voice of Roger Waters.

I marched down Broad Street till I reached 5 Corners, one of those fucked up intersections that sprang up out of the dirt in the 18th Century when three or four farm roads converge just on what was then the outskirts of the 'city.' I took a left onto Queen Street, which is really a misnomer, unless the queen it was named after (Liz the First) was an alcoholic and drug addict.

Queen Street divided one of the best parts of town, and one of the worst. It was an amazing border between the Historic District of a very old town and the place where you can find anything you want, providing what you want is prostitution, crack-cocaine, or some kind of disease that will rot off your penis and testicles. On the left side, the west side of Queen Street were the 'projects,' i.e., government housing for the poorest of the poor. It was a hot-bed of crime and misery.

Half the way down Queen Street was the police station, which was appropriate and ironic, all at the same time, because behind the station was the Frog Pond convenient store, *convenient* if you are in need of a whore, some crack, or a disease that will rot off your private parts. Behind 'The Pond', as we referred to it, was an alleyway. From that alleyway, you could see the back wall of the police station, a brick edifice which for some reason had no windows on that side. If there *had* been windows, every cop in New Bern could have witnessed all the crimes they were sworn to protect the citizens against, in full swing.

Of course, the cops knew that all this was going on, and did very little to stop it. Someone was getting greased, that's for sure, and probably very high up. Because if *I* knew what was going on behind The Pond, New Bern's Finest could not reasonably claim ignorance.

I strolled past The Pond and the police station, which were on the other side of the street from me. I didn't want to interact with either of those groups of people. I had no intention of ordering off the menu at The Pond — no thank you — or hanging out with a bunch of cops with a fifth of liquor in my hand. I continued on down the street, and glanced over at Cedar Grove Cemetery, where I used to do lawn care. It was a reminder of all I'd lost, and so a constant negative influence on my mind; I had to walk past it, every fuckin' day.

As I was passing the limestone walls and gateway of Cedar Grove, I heard the footsteps.

This wasn't abnormal; I was on a public sidewalk, after all. But my Spidey Senses began to tingle for some reason. I suppose they were always on alert when I was walking home in that part of town. But I had a fifth of liquor in my hands, which suggested to anyone on the street that I had just been paid, and that made me a target.

I suddenly felt like one. The hairs on my arm stood up.

I picked up speed. This was a natural, *Lizard Brain* Fear reaction. It was also a test. It was very much like a movie scene. Someone is being followed, so they start walking faster to see if the person behind does the same. But whatever you do, you don't look back. Hell no. That would signal that you're afraid and leave you very vulnerable.

Whoever was behind me sped up, too.

At that point, I was pretty sure they were following me, and since they hadn't yelled out my name, that meant only one thing; they had evil intentions and I was in trouble.

It was then that I heard the whispering voices. There were at least two of them.

Fuck.

I didn't dare look back, though it was a fight not to.

I sped up even more.

They matched it, and were gaining on me. I could hear it.

They were getting closer by the second.

At this point, I was about to pass the Salvation Army church and Thrift Store on the other side of the street. On my right, my side of the street, was a one story apartment complex, probably built in the 60s, because it was ugly as fuck like everything built in that decade. Between the back wall of that building and the sidewalk where I was walking quickly, was a grassy area, maybe 20 feet wide, with a grouping of pine trees dotting the yard.

Just as I was passing this building, I saw, out of the corner of my right eye, one of the *gentlemen* — and I use that term very fuckin' loosely — sweeping out amongst the trees, attempting to get an *angle* on me: essentially, a flanking maneuver. The blood ran to my ears, my heart was pounding in my chest, and I prepared to run.

I heard one quick step behind me.

Whoever it was, was breaking into a run.

I was gone.

In that instant, there were three things I could have done. I could have frozen in Fear: not a good option. I could have turned to fight them off: also not good, since I was outnumbered and had no weapon, other than the bottle of whiskey that I had no intention of giving up. So, I chose Door Number Three: run like fuckin' hell.

I kicked in the nitrous overdrive, dropped it into 2nd gear and veered into the street. I went from four or five miles per hour, walking, to 100 mph running, in about one-tenth of a second.

As I hit the middle of the street, I heard them running, too. And then a glass bottle sailed past my left ear and smashed in the street.

Another one buzzed my right ear, crashing into the pavement on my right.

I was in full-on, Lizard Brain flight mode at this point. There was no thought of fight.

I ran.

I ran like a muthafucker.

I don't know for sure who was behind me, but I do know

something: whoever it was, I guarantee you they had never seen a white boy run so fast.

I was only a block from home at that point, and I covered the distance at warp speed, sole-less shoes, bare feet, polyester costume, bottle of whiskey, and all.

The next day, I walked into K-Mart—yeah, that's how old this story is—and purchased a very sharp, fishing filet knife. (When Patience read this sentence, she wrote in the margins, "Why didn't you get new shoes? Which is a logical question, for which I have no logical answer. I plead the stupidity of youth.)

The knife had a wooden handle, and a long, thin, blade that would have laid open a dragon, if you could get close enough to shove it in between its scales. I put that thing on a belt, and I wore it to work every day until I was fired from that job for eating a chicken tender. I wore that knife right out where everyone could see it, just in case some dumbass decided to chase me again, or follow me home. The next time, they'd get a fight, not a flight.

FEAR AS A GIFT: PROTECTION FROM DANGER?

"Planning for the future is only ever useful to those who know how to fully live in the present." —Alan Watts

What was my purpose in sharing this story, other than the fact that it's a great example of fight or flight Fear?

I think that it works on a couple of levels.

One, it's fight or flight. But it's easy to come up with those stories. We all have them. So what?

The significance, for this book, is that my Lizard Brain Fear saved my ass from a mugging that day. As soon as I heard the footsteps behind me I knew something was up. Something wasn't quite right about those steps, about the whispered voices, about the way their speed kept matching mine. I *knew* that they were up to no good, blocks before they broke into a run behind me. My instincts, *Fear* instincts, warned me of the attack, long before it happened.

Can Fear be a Gift?

Author Gavin de Becker, in *The Gift of Fear*, suggests that Fear is a gift, and I would have to agree that it is, sometimes.

De Becker claims that he's spent most of this life living in the future, trying to predict possible violent acts before they occur. I'm not quite convinced—on the future part of it, anyway. In a certain sense, I suppose he *is* correct; the acts have not occurred, therefore, part of his mind is in the future imagining what will happen if his predictions are off. But the predictions themselves, the clues that lead him to those predictions, exist in only two places: the past and the present.

He can draw from past experiences, thousands of them in his case, to help him predict what people *might* do. But in order to predict what will happen in the immediate future, he absolutely *must* focus on the NOW, the present moment, or he would miss all of the micro clues that drive his intuition.

I think that when de Becker speaks of Fear existing only in the future, he's drawing a very sharp line between the *now* and the *soon to be*. I'm more inclined to think of an *expansive* present, or as Alan Watts might call it, an eternal present, though I wouldn't push it quite to that extent for the purposes of discussing Fear.

I think it's more helpful to think of the present, not as something that is only momentary—a fleeting snap of the fingers, here and gone again in a flash—but as having space on either side of that snappy, flashy instant.

One of the examples that de Becker uses to illustrate this point is one where we are sitting in our living room, with a Fear that one day, or night, a thief might burst through our plate-glass window. That Fear exists only in the future because, as de Becker argues, it hasn't yet happened. For de Becker, all Fear exists only in the future, as an anticipation of some dangerous event.

Once the thief *actually* breaks into our living room we no longer have a Fear of that, de Becker argues. Instead, we now shift our Fears to what might happen *next*; will the thief pull out a gun and kill us or just steal our stereo? These things have not yet happened, and as such, are in the future.

While the thief hasn't pulled his pistol, I think it's fair to say that the incident is *ongoing*, and therefore, still in the present. What

I think Mr. de Becker and I *would* agree upon is that the Fear we are feeling is *occurring* in the present, as it always is. Nothing occurs in the past or the future. They are, for all intents and purposes, no-man's lands; they don't really exist. One doesn't exist anymore and the other never does.

All *experiences* we have of the past and the future occur *only* in the present.

A Gift, but Only If

I think the most important point that de Gavin presents in his book is that our Fears of what *might* happen in the future can cripple our intuition and instincts in the present. Most of our Fears *do* reside in a Future-land where we never really live. If we are focused on those illusions, we might miss the footsteps on the pavement behind us and end up another statistic.

Without focus on the present, the past is useless and the future becomes more dangerous, and quite frankly, pointless.

Alan Watts, the eminent 20th Century, hippie-philosopher, once said, "Planning for the future is only ever useful to those who know how to fully live in the present." And that is what is at the heart of this book. It is my attempt to help us eliminate all the useless Fears so that we can actually live in the present.

Sometimes, that means being afraid, or fearing, listening to our Lizard Brain intuition, so that we can avoid danger. But mostly, it's so that we can live in peace, friendship, and prosperity *now*, instead of worrying constantly about the future. If we eliminate those future Fears, then we can be in the now, avoid danger more easily and live a fuller life.

But no matter how useful Fear can be in certain situations, if our minds are preoccupied with irrelevant, senseless Fears, it will be unable to discern the difference between a *real threat*—like a mugger, a rapist, or murderous husband—and just something we *perceive* to be a real threat—the pain of losing our midnight, Twinkie Eating Fest, if we go on that diet that we're dreading. More often than not, our instincts are overridden by insignificant Fears. And *that* is the real threat because then our Lizard Brain can't function in the way it was designed.

If I had ignored my instincts that day walking down Queen Street and failed to run because I might look stupid, or chicken shit, then I might have gotten my ass kicked, lost my Traveller's Club Whiskey, and ended up in the hospital, or worse. But in *that* situation, I listened to my Lizard and I survived.

What's also significant about that incident, beyond the attempted mugging, was my subsequent reaction; I bought a weapon. I wore it openly as a warning. It was meant to instill Fear into anyone with ill intentions. I ramped up the Fear, in other words. I was fighting a very real threat with a threat of my own.

This was taking my Fear to a new level: what I call Monkey Brain Fear and *Homo sapiens* Fear: Fears that live in the past and the future.

When confronted with a real threat, we remember it, and then project similar threats into the future to prepare for them. Sometimes this is useful, but we almost always carry it too far. Carrying our reaction too far leads to an escalation of Fear, which rarely leads to good things. In fact, de Becker contends that this uber-vigilance actually undermines and clouds our instincts, making us *more* vulnerable, not less; and I agree.

My logical Fear of actually being mugged turned into a Known Fear, an event in the past; I had been chased. I then took that historic moment and projected it into the future —*I will probably be chased or mugged, again* —and I prepared for it. I bought a knife and displayed it for all to see, as a warning: *don't fuck with me, or you'll lose your guts*. I graduated from true *victim* of Fear and violence, to a *perpetuator* of Fear, threatening violence.

How else could I have responded?

Well, I could have reasoned that I'd only been chased once, and therefore it wasn't all that likely that it would happen again. That wouldn't have been a safe assumption, not given the neighborhood that I was walking through. There were all sorts of unsavory types on that route.

I could have chosen a different route to come home. There weren't a lot of options, but I could have walked a couple blocks past Queen Street, and then turned to walk through the Historic District, which was safer, for sure. But that would have been giving in to Fear in a different way. I would have allowed my perceived Fear—that of being mugged—to dictate where and when I would go.

That rankled me. *Fuck that* was my thought. *I'll go wherever I want!* But that's a different kind of Fear: the Fear of the Loss of Identity, i.e., my John Wayne manhood. More on that later.

To be fair to those who advocate that we should all carry weapons, I was never attacked again. But who knows what my reaction set off in other directions? I will never know.

So, can Fear be a Gift?

Yes, sometimes.

If you're afraid of crossing the street, you might look left, then right, then left again before stepping off the curb. Or maybe you see a hairy, shirtless man walking down the street, wearing a kilt, swinging a broadsword. It might pay to give me a wide berth, especially if I don't have a cold drink in my hand and there's steam coming off my head. Being afraid in those situations might be a good idea, and help to keep you around another day. But most of the Fears we have aren't keeping us alive or out of danger; they're killing us, one razor cut at a time, and we don't even know it.

Worse than that, we may be afraid of the very opportunities that could launch us to the success that we crave so badly. When Opportunity comes a knockin', it's not always dressed in a Santa Suit. Sometimes it comes disguised as a Land Shark singing telegram. (*If you didn't get that reference to the ancient Saturday Night Live skit, look it up.*)

While Fear can sometimes help us to avoid very nasty situations, it can also lead us into a land of illusion, where we begin to think that there really *is* a thing called safety.

Is Safety an Illusion?

"The Fear of Death follows from the Fear of Life. A man who lives fully is prepared to die at any time." —Mark Twain

"Gomer! Get that gun out'cha mouth!" —Sheriff Andy Taylor, *Andy Griffith Show*

How do we know that being realistic, or following our Fears, will keep us out of danger?

I don't think we can.

No one knows the Future. Any one of us could die of a heart attack right now, fall down the stairs and break our neck, or be crushed in a flaming car crash this afternoon. There IS no safety. It is *all* illusion.

Are Some Situations Safer Than Others?

Sure. Sitting in my home office, in my overstuffed chair is probably safer than charging through Afghanistan with an American Flag on my back. Just as NOT kissing a cobra is safer than kissing one, and not putting the end of a shotgun in your mouth is safer than doing it. All these things are true.

But to argue that taking one job over another, turning left instead of right at the intersection, or *not* following your intuition and passion to do what you want to do is safer than *doing* it is absurd in the extreme—unless of course your passion is to run through a terrorist camp wearing Old Glory with a gun in your mouth, stopping to kiss some cobras on the way—not something I'd advise you to attempt.

Fear doesn't guarantee safety; nothing does.

Fear is mostly just killing us at 25, rendering us into rotting, walking corpses, long before they throw the dust on us and say the fuckin' prayers. There's a far greater risk to not taking risks, I would argue, and that is the risk of *not* doing what we want: the risk of being realistic.

THE DANGER OF BEING REALISTIC: ON THE ROAD TO A ZOMBIELAND

"A single dream is more powerful than a thousand realities." — Nathaniel Hawthorne

How do we know that not taking a risk to follow our dreams isn't actually riskier?

What about the road you *didn't* take?

How do you know that sitting still is safer than moving? Fire and maneuver my friend. Sitting still is death. Just ask any veteran about that one. How do we know that being afraid is less risky than being courageous?

We can't know because the answers are in a future that we can never see because it doesn't exist, and never will.

All we can do is right now

We can act, or not act, both of which are decisions. Don't think for a second that you're putting off making a decision by choosing not to do something. Choosing *is* a decision, and every choice comes with unforeseen consequences: every one. And you have no idea what those are going to be.

Wouldn't it be better, for the sake of our life's story to say that when faced with decisions we just *chose* and moved on? We sucked up courage in the face of Fear, spat in that bastard's eye, and did what we wanted to do? Is that not a better choice than cowering in your easy chair, wishing and wondering what your life might be like if you could only find a *safe* way to achieve your dreams?

There are no *safe* paths, just paths. So choose one, and go!

Reality, Mediocrity, and Zombies

Fear creates its own false reality, a negative one, which attracts more of the same. Such a *reality* is simply an excuse for mediocrity.

To give into our Fear is to doom ourselves to the path of mediocrity because it tricks us into abandoning our dreams.

And if we give up on our dreams, are we not already dead? Many people give up on their dreams at 25, die inside, and live the rest of their miserable lives waiting around to be buried at 80. They are zombies, in the real sense of the word.

Fear drives this insanity and it creates a box of so-called *reality*, which traps us. Fuck the box! Burn the box down and toss the ashes to the wind! *Realism* is for the weak. *Safety* is for the weak. And they are both illusions.

The absolute truth is that we create our *own* reality. To give into a reality that says we should remain in a safe box is to surrender to mediocrity. Nothing great was ever created by being *realistic* or *mediocre*. Sir Isaac Newton, Thomas Edison, Albert Einstein, Steve Jobs, and Mahatma Gandhi all have one thing in common; they ignored *reality*, ignored *mediocrity*, and created *new* realities. If you aren't doing the same, why not?

Fear is why.

Is Fear a Useful Motivator?

Something in the grass, moved.

My heart jumped and then sank.

My hands went cold.

I froze in my tracks, if standing in ten inches of river water counts as *tracks*. The gas trimmer was humming and vibrating in my hands, the stainless steel blade at the end of the tool singing a high-pitched whine; the whole thing vibrated violently in my hands, as I stared down through the tall marsh grass into the dark water.

Between the blades of green, I saw two eyes.

In 1988, I was 22 years old, recently married, and the father of a beautiful little girl. I was also broke and desperate to make money. I had been working for my father at the Salvation Army in New Bern, NC, for a couple of years. While the job was okay, it didn't pay enough to support a wife and child.

Working along with me, was our youth director from the church, Ken. The two of us cooked up a plan one day, after driving past Cedar Grove Cemetery, to start up a new business: landscaping and lawncare. The cemetery had potential to be a showplace, but in 1988, it was overgrown and a bit derelict. The city was struggling to keep the place up.

Long story short, we borrowed some equipment and convinced the city that were were the men for the job, and off we went into the Land of Scaping.

But I digress.

You want to know about the black eyes in the dark water.

That summer, Ken and I busted ass and created a little business for ourselves, enough of one that a couple of months into it, we both quit working at the Salvation Army. We were cutting grass and doing landscaping all over the city. One of the jobs we took that summer was down in the country club area, on the Trent River, a fresh water river which flows into the Neuse River where the city of New Bern was founded back in 1710. And that's how I ended up standing in ten inches of marsh grass in the Trent River, staring at a pair of black eyes.

We were hired by an old guy—who had an overpriced, ranch-style home on the river—to come in and cut down all of his marsh grass so he could better see the river. Now, trust me, this isn't something I would do *now*. I'm much too environmentally conscious these days. But back then, I wasn't. I was *economically* conscious: conscious of the fact that I didn't have any money and a daughter and wife at home to feed. So, we took the job. I'm not even sure it was legal to do what we did.

Now, you have to realize that when I say some marsh grass, I mean a patch of grass reaching out into the river about 50 yards, and probably 70 yards wide! It was a huge area to cut, and it couldn't be accomplished with a riding mower! It had to be cut down, one swath at a time, with the swing of a weed-whipper.

The grass was very thick, close to an inch at the water level, so the standard weed-whipper string wasn't gonna get'er done. We had to attach our brush-blade: a ten-inch, stainless steel blade that could instantly whack down a small tree of an inch or two in diameter. It was more than capable of taking down the marsh grass, and it did so with ease. The only problem with the blade is that it caused the whole machine to vibrate in a very uncomfortable way. You could feel the vibrations all the way up your arm, and after using the tool for 5 or 10 minutes you had to pry your hands off of it because your fingers would freeze in position.

We arrived the morning of the job and Ken took first duty on the whipper. We did at least have one pair of fishing boots to wade in the water. He pulled them on and dove into the job. After slogging around in the water for about 30 minutes along the shore, he decided he wanted to cut the job in half, so he began to cut a path straight through the middle of the patch of grass, out to the river.

Slowly but surely, he managed to do just that.

That's when he stepped in a sinkhole of mud.

His left foot and leg disappeared in a second, and he almost went under the water.

He yelled to me for help, "Steeeeve! I can't pull my leg out!"

But I was standing on the shore in tennis shoes! There was no second set of boots; we were running on a very small budget. So, I had to run out to him, through the muddy water, in tennis shoes, to pull him out of a hole!

So I did.

I managed to get to him, pull him out, sans the one boot, which he then reached down to retrieve, and we both sloshed our way back up to shore, exhausted.

He then announced that it was *my turn* to take over. I reluctantly agreed.

Ken took off to go price another job on the other side of town and left me alone to keep working, with the promise he'd be back shortly.

I cranked up the whipper, the blade singing in the hot, sticky, Southern air, and waded out into the water, swinging my weapon before me.

I hadn't gone more than 20 feet, I think, when something moved in the water about 10 feet in front of me. That's when I stopped in my soggy tracks.

Whatever it was, was about the size of a very large bullfrog. It had eyes—very dark ones—that were staring up at me.

And then it moved.

It didn't hop.

Frogs hop.

Toads hop.

But this didn't fuckin' hop.

It *slid* forward.

It slid forward an inch, or two, and stopped, staring me straight in the eye. The hair on my arms stood up, my heart raced, my sweat turned icy cold, and I froze in place. I was mesmerized by those eyes. I was looking in to the face of a cold-blooded killer.

I was face to face with Mr. No-Shoulders: a watermoccasin, and a very big one at that. His head was the size of a dessert plate, maybe six or seven inches in diameter. Later, when I was able to think about such things, I estimated that he must have been 15 to 20 feet long. But I never saw the body of Mr. No-Shoulders. All I ever saw was the head. The rest was hidden in the dark, muddy water of the river.

I stood, fixed in place, Fear running through every nerve in my body, oozing out of my pores and freezing my mind. I couldn't think. I was too afraid to think, at least for several seconds. We both stood, staring at each other, the weed-whipper singing its steely song. All I could think was something that some old-timer once told me about snakes, *"If you see one, you can bet there's another ten ya* don't *see."*

And that thought roused me from my hypnosis and broke the spell of those black eyes.

Then everything was a blurr.

I smacked the steel blade down into the water in front of me, daring Mr. No-Shoulders to come!

He didn't.

He slid back into the water, which should have given me some sense of relief, but it occasioned an opposite reaction.

The motion of that snake slipping backward and disappearing into the water, was one of the scariest things I've ever seen, because then, I couldn't *see* him at all! He had instantly moved from a *known* Fear, one I could see and size up, to an *unknown* one, lurking somewhere in the water, waiting for me to return.

I did the only thing my terrified mind would allow me to do.

I turned to flight.

I did *not* stand to fight.

I got the hell out of that water as fast as I could move, all the while smacking the blade of the whipper down into the water to scare off any children, spouses, or cousins of the No-Shoulders family!

I made it to shore in a couple of seconds. I was standing there, my heart thumping in my ears, sweat running into my eyes and the whipper still vibrating violently in my hands.

I managed to get my right hand free even though it was mostly frozen in place. Then I managed to pry my left hand free of the handle after pushing the kill switch on the machine.

I was a wreck.

I was shaking with Fear.

I stood there, looking out at all of that marsh grass, and all I could see was hundreds of water-moccasins, swirling around under that fuckin' muddy water, just waiting for me to return so they could fill me full of venom.

I sat down on the red-brick steps at the back of the house, the whipper at my feet, silent as the grave. The crickets were humming and sawing their wings in the background. You could *hear* the heat of that Southern summer. But all I could really hear was my own heart slamming in my ears, and the stinging numbness of my hands.

I sat there, for probably 30 minutes or more debating with myself and with my Fear. I was definitely afraid. I'd never liked snakes: still don't. I realize they have their place in the ecosystem so I give them that. But that day, the snake stood between me and the money I desperately needed to feed and shelter my family. If it weren't for that desperation, Mr. No-Shoulders would have won the debate: no doubt whatsoever about that one.

But I needed that money.

How could I go home to my wife and tell her that I gave up on a customer, and therefore, wouldn't be able to pay the rent or buy groceries?

There was no fuckin' way I was gonna do *that*. I'd rather face a whole *family* of No-Shoulders than face my ex-wife with *that* kind of news. If you think staring down a snake is tough, try staring down my ex. Some Fears trump other Fears, and that is a lesson to remember.

After a long debate with my Fear on that hot, sticky day in 1988, I picked up my weed-whipper, pulled the starter cord, and I waded back out into that river. You can bet that I plunged that singing blade into the water at every step! I made sure that if any of Mr. No-Shoulder's cousins were still around, that they knew I meant business, and that I would cut them into little fuckin' pieces if they so much as reared their slimy heads! I didn't see any more of them that day and neither did Ken, once he returned. But I've never forgotten that day and the Fear I felt while staring into those black eyes.

What do you Fear more than the Fear in front of you?

In my case, the Fears of Scarcity, Poverty, Failure, Criticism, my own perceived Inadequacies, and my wife's disappointment, tipped the scales on my Fear of the entire species of No-Shoulders.

Fear can most certainly be a powerful motivator.

But is it a good one?

In the past, I've often proposed that it was, but I'm not so sure anymore.

Supposedly, it kicks us in the ass to get out of bed, go to work, make more money, get a better job, and therefore, not to starve to death or be thrown out into the street to suffer the ravages of the environment, as it did for me that day in the marsh grass.

It is our survival instinct. We are motivated to move because we're afraid of what will happen if we don't: Scarcity, Poverty,

Failure, Criticism, and a bunch of other Fears.

There's something to this train of thought, but we carry it too far. Yes, it is our instinct to get up and get moving in order to obtain food, water, shelter, etc. That is something inherent in all animals. But I don't think Fear of annihilation, or death, or starvation, is a particularly *great* motivator. It motivates, for sure, but I think there are much better reasons to pick our ass up off the couch every day.

Instinct Over-Ride: Burying the Gift of Fear

The most dangerous thing about Fear as a motivator is that it motivates us to do the wrong thing at the wrong time, in the wrong way.

This is illustrated well in the story of Mr. No-Shoulders.

My instincts for survival, my basic Fear, told me to get the fuck out of the water and not go back! But my Fears of what might happen if I didn't, over-rode what Gavin de Becker called the Gift of Fear, my instincts, and I waded back out into that poisonous, snake-infested water where there was a *real threat* to life and limb: a water-moccasin the size of Texas.

Death was a very real possibility in that water. As much as it might have *felt* deadly to go home and face my wife without that money, I'm fairly certain that death would not have been the result. My Fears of the consequences were mostly illusions. Yes, I would have passed up on some money. But what if Mr. No-Shoulders had decided to defend his watery house? The cost of my funeral would have been much higher than my pay.

This is what de Becker warns us about in his book. If we allow our irrational Fears to control us, we will do some pretty stupid shit, like dancing around with poisonous snakes, or following wolfish abusive husbands into the woods.

So, does Fear motivate us?

Yes, it does.

Is that a good thing?

Fuck no, it isn't.

There's only one way in which our Fears can have a positive effect; they can inspire us to be courageous in the face of them.

TRIGGER FOR COURAGE AND COMMUNITY

Can Fear trigger *positive* responses?

Yes. In challenging, scary, and dangerous circumstances it can trigger one of the most powerful responses: courage.

We'll talk more about courage later in the book, but I want to say now, that if something fearful happens and your reaction is to be courageous and face it then the act of fearing served a very good purpose. Fear and courage have a very interesting relationship; one can have Fear without courage, but not courage without Fear. Courage, one of the most positive emotions and mindsets, is wholly dependent upon the existence of Fear, or at least fear*ing*. A little fearing can be a good thing if our response is courage.

We've all witnessed acts of courage in our lives. Most of us have probably performed courageous acts. They're not always saving children from burning buildings, diving into frozen rivers to save kittens, or landing jumbo jets on a tarmac without the proper wheels. It might be something as simple as walking on stage to give a short speech, asking for that raise you've deserved for ten years, or facing your wife to tell her you walked away from money in order to not be injected with deadly moccasin venom. Those are courageous acts, too.

And we're going to need all the courage we can muster, as we return to the dark Forest of Fear. This time, we're going to spend some time camping under the black shadows of the Father of the Forest: the Tree of Fear Itself.

GOODIE BASKET THREE: A TRICKY GIFT

- **Our instinctual**, Lizard Brain Fear *can* be a gift to keep us safer in potentially dangerous situations.

- **Fear Itself**, however, can override our instincts, leading us to do really stupid, dangerous things.

- If we choose to **face our Fears with courage**, then they have served some purpose.

4

One Big-Assed Tree

ARE THERE TOO MANY FEARS?

"Actually ... they were not far off the edge of the forest; and if Bilbo had had the sense to see it, the tree that he had climbed, though it was tall in itself, was standing near the bottom of a wide valley, so that from its top the trees seemed to swell up all around like the edges of a great bowl, and he could not expect to see how far the forest lasted. Still he did not see this, and he climbed down full of despair."
—J.R.R. Tolkien, *The Hobbit*

If you can remember back to the Introduction of this book, we listed the Five Myths about the World's Problems. The fourth one on that list was that there were just *too many Fears* to count, and that the topic was too complicated and complex to ever sort it all out. There are just too many branches, twigs, leaves, and fruit on the Tree of Fear.

At first glance, hell, even after weeks of thinking about it, I would have agreed with you. But my brain works in a peculiar way. It loves to take complex problems and try to make them simple. And the more I began to look at the topic of Fear, the more I thought, *"There must be a way to break all of these down into simpler themes, or categories.*

And that's essentially what psychologists, clinical psychologists at least, have traditionally been doing: cataloging our Fears and other mental disorders. While there's some limited use to listing them all—maybe—the limits are narrow and serve very little purpose in addressing the problems caused by Fear. This is just enumerating and attempting to treat *symptoms* instead of looking for the roots of the problem.

Fear tends to pop up everywhere. If we tried to attack every single way that it comes into our lives, all the nasty fruits of the Tree, this book would swell to many thousands of pages and probably create it's own category of Fear: the *Fear of Being Crushed by One of Steve Bivans's Books*.

Instead, let's see if we can group them into some larger categories. I call them the *branches*, the *trunk*, and the *roots*. Then we'll cut that damned Tree down to size and come up with broad strategies and tactics that will apply to all the daily instances of Fear that grow on the gnarly twigs.

The Anatomy of the Tree of Fear

I'm quite certain that numerous authors, psychologists, and life coaches have proposed categories of Fear, but since I haven't read them all, and it would take too long anyway, I'm going to focus on two that I've come across, and then try to boil them down into what I think are the main categories of Fear.

The first guy who tried to tackle the categories of Fear was Napoleon Hill, in his 1930s book, *Think and Grow Rich*. According to Hill, our Fears are a major blocker when it comes to achieving our goals, be they monetary—as he was most concerned with—or otherwise. He was correct, of course. Fears really *are* roadblocks to any kind of success.

Hill proposed that there were six categories of major fears:

1. Fear of Death
2. Fear of Old Age
3. Fear of Criticism
4. Fear of Ill Health
5. Fear of Loss of Love
6. Fear of Poverty

I think some of these fall into larger categories, but we'll look at that in a minute.

Brendon Burchard, one of the most popular life coaches alive today, has proposed that there are only three categories.

Burchard's are based on the Fear of Pain:

1. Fear of the Pain of Loss
2. Fear of the Pain of Process
3. Fear of the Pain of Outcome

Pain of Loss is pretty self explanatory, and I believe things like health and life and death fall within those, as well as loss of love.

Pain of Process simply means the sacrifices and energy that we

have to expend to achieve, or attempt to achieve, some goal, whether that be losing weight, making money, changing jobs, getting a divorce, etc.

Pain of Outcome simply means that we fear the ultimate outcome of our efforts, in other words, will we be successful? Will we fail?

I think Mr. Hill, and Mr. Burchard have both presented some interesting ideas, but Hill's are too diffuse—some of them fit into tighter categories—and Burchard has left out three that I think don't fit into any of his.

Here are all but one of the categories of Fear, as I see them:
1. Fear of the Pain of Outcome
2. Fear of the Pain of Process
3. Fear of the Pain of Loss
4. Fear of the Known
5. Fear of the Unknown

There's one more major Fear, one I think is the seed of the entire, deadly Tree, but we'll get to it in time. First, let's examine the others in more detail.

I'm going to do something curious in our examination. Instead of beginning with the seed and roots of the Tree of Fear, I'm gonna start with the branches and fruits.

There's a method to my madness, I assure you, so hang on. We're going *fruits* to *roots*. Hope you brought a sturdy tent, because camping under this Tree can get pretty icky.

Limbs, Leaves, and Fruit: Living in the Canopy of Our Future Fears

"Fear is not real. The only place that fear can exist is in our thoughts of the future. It is a product of our imagination, causing us to fear things that

do not at present and may not ever exist. That is near insanity. Do not misunderstand me danger is very real but fear is a choice." —Will Smith, actor and supreme ass kicker

One of the biggest problems I ran into at the beginning of this project was to make sense of the seemingly endless Fears that we all encounter. This is especially true of the three categories that I would call the *branches* of the Tree of Fear that Brenden Burchard suggested: Fear of the Pain of Loss, Pain of Process, and Pain of Outcome.

These are what I would call *projected*, or irrational, Fears. They are the ones that most of us can identify: the ones we all know and deal with every day. If I were to ask you what your major Fears were, you would probably give me a list of *projected Fears*, the *fruits* of the Tree. You might hit on some Fears from the branches, maybe even the trunk, but probably not much deeper unless you've given it a lot of thought before.

From Fruit to Root

I want to start with the *fruits* at the top of the Tree, because I want to work backwards, or downwards, from what you *know* to what you might not be aware of. The problem with trying to explain complex ideas is that they can never be explained, fully, with the use of language. Words are just inadequate to describe the world around us, and that's a bold statement coming from an author.

For instance, do you know how your entire body works? Your body and all of its systems work all by themselves, every day, without your conscious thought. You don't have to *think* about your heart beat, unless it goes all wonky or stops completely. It just keeps beating. You don't have to tell your brain to *think*. You don't have to tell your lungs to breathe. They just do it. It isn't really complicated or complex. It's only complicated if you attempt to explain it to someone else, in words. Even if you're a surgeon, it's impossible to explain all the things that are happening in the human body in a way that can be understood by the average person, or even another surgeon.

I won't give you a brain aneurism, or stop your heart with a belabored and boring discussion of the limitations of language. Suffice it to say that it isn't the *functioning* of Fear that is complex, only the *explanation* that makes it complicated.

So, what I'm going to attempt to do with words (or what I am already attempting to do, since you're half way through the book by now) is to *un*explain Fear. That is, take it from the most complicated manifestations, down to the simplest. To use our running tree metaphor, I'm going to take you from the fruit to the root. The root is very simple: ridiculously simple, in fact. The fruit? Complicated as hell. But if I can demonstrate how all of those fruits connect to major branches of the Tree of Fear, then they become less complicated.

Living in the Canopy of Our Future Fears

Most of us live the vast majority of our lives in a place that doesn't exist: the future.

And the only reason we do it is because Fear tells us that's where we should be. It tells us that the present doesn't exist; it's a snap of the fingers.

Most of us recall Fears from past negative experiences. Since these events still haunt us, causing pain and suffering, we are deathly afraid that we will encounter such experiences again in the Future. We take those Fears and project them into the future, either the immediate future, or days, weeks, months, years ahead. This is when our Fears become really nasty and destructive.

The future doesn't exist; it never will. It exists only in our minds as an image of what we want it to be, or more often than not, what we *don't* want it to be. But by focusing on what we don't want, we usually get it. Okay, we *always* get it.

Thought Is Reality

The mind is a powerful thing. It creates our reality, every day, throughout our lives. Perception really *is* reality, because what we *think* is reality, *is* our reality. It matters not that it isn't everyone else's reality. In the end, only our reality matters to us. But it isn't an external reality; it's our own creation. We may have some *help* in creating it; things *do* happen *to* us. But we choose how we want to frame those experiences, 100 percent.

The future doesn't exist but we act as if it does. Life exists in only one place, the present. When we project our Fears into the future we destroy the present, the only time we truly have.

Our most ancient ancestors, our lizard grandparents, had very small brains, really just a brain *stem*, which was only good for recognizing threats in the present. Our more recent ancestors, Granny and Pa Ape, developed a more complex brain, what we'll call our Monkey Brain, which could record events from the past, helping them better recognize potential threats in the present.

But as the brains of our ancestors developed ever more complexity, the complexity of our Fears grew along with them. Eventually we developed the frontal lobe of the brain, which marked our shift to *Homo sapiens*. When that happened, we were able not only to perceive immediate threats and remember threats from our past, but to postulate that there might be threats in this new, unknown territory called the future. The future did not exist as an idea until we developed our frontal lobe.

Once we had this new appendage, we could take past threats and Fears, and project them into the future to avoid such encounters with lions, tigers, and bears. Eventually, we were able to make plans for the future that would better ensure our survival and the survival of our species. Once this occurred, we began to multiply the number of possible threats and Fears and the game was on.

Part of planning for the future is to analyze and minimize the risks, whether that is the likelihood of encountering lions, tigers, and bears or the possibility that we will lose all of our savings in a Wall Street crash. Once we analyze them, and if we think a particular outcome is likely, we project those Fears into the future as if it's already occurred.

Next, we're going to take a look at some of the ways in which we project Fear by gathering them together into Brendon Burchard's three categories, the *branches* — Loss, Process, and Outcome. By giving some examples of how those Fears manifest themselves in our lives, you'll be able to recognize each category, if not in your own life, then in the actions of people you know.

We're going to start with a dangling limb, the Widow Maker: the Fear of the Pain of Loss.

Under a Hanging Branch: The Widow-Maker & the Fear of Pain of Loss

"There is nothing that is so much the very essence of suffering, as the Fear of Suffering Itself."

—Alan Watts, 20th century Philosophical Entertainer and Zen

Hippie Bad Ass

I have a vague childhood memory of walking through a Forest with an old person — which probably means they were like, you know, 30 something — and walking under an old tree which sported a rotten, hanging branch of some large size, dangling precariously above my head.

"Don't stand under that!" the old person said, "It's a Widow-Maker!"

I stared up at his ancient face, with a strange look on my face. I hadn't heard him correctly.

"Window Maker?" I asked in my little boy voice. I don't actually remember having a little boy voice, but I'm sure I must have at some point, back when the Earth was still cooling.

"No! Wid-OW-Maker!" he replied.

"What's a Wid-OW?"

"It's a woman who has lost her husband." he said.

"Oh" I said, still obviously confused.

He could tell that the term still eluded me, or at least how it connected to dangling branches. I wasn't quite as learn*ed* as I am now. Maybe this was my first lesson in practical metaphor-ing; I'm not sure.

"If the limb falls on your head, you'll be dead," he explained in rhyme, "and your wife will be a widow!"

"OHHHH!" And that was a moment of enlightenment. I've never walked through a Forest since without noticing the Widow-Makers.

The Fear of the Pain of Loss is like a dangling branch over our heads. It could fall at any time, and take something, or someone, away from us forever. It's an unsettling, painful thought.

We all have a Fear of losing something, usually a whole long list of somethings. At the base of this is a Fear of losing our own life or the lives of the people we care about. But this branch of the Tree includes many other forms of loss. A short list would include loss of love, money, security, food, wealth, pleasure, comfort, reputation, and status.

Let's return to our Land of Oz analogy and imagine you're strolling down the Yellow Brick Road with your mother-in-law. Would you really mind if a lion, tiger, or bear carried her off? It might just make your day!

If I were to lose 100 pounds of body fat, for instance, I would not have a Fear of that. I would be happier than a pig in shit.

The Fear of the Pain of Loss is also one of our ancestors' earliest Fears: probably Monkey Brain stuff. While time and space won't allow us to catalogue every fruit on this branch, there are a few sub-categories of Loss that we should examine, because they are common and illustrate the power of this Fear.

FEAR OF DEATH

"It is not death that a man should fear, but he should fear never beginning to live." — Marcus Aurelius, Roman emperor, philosopher, and super cool dude in a toga

Our oldest Fear is most likely the Fear of Death.

This is, of course, also a Fear of the Unknown. We don't know what really happens when we die and we also don't know the manner in which our death will occur. Will we suffer? Will our loved ones suffer? We want them to be around forever. To lose them leaves a massive hole in our emotional mind.

This one Fear underlies many of our others. Even the Fear of the Pain of Outcome, an entire category of Fears, is built upon this one. The Fear of Failure — one of the major outcome Fears is firmly rooted in the Fear of Loss. What do we really fear when we fail? Mainly, that we will lose something, or a lot of things, if we aren't successful at our job, at parenting, at whatever.

The Fear of our own death, or that of our family members, significant others, friends, or even neighbors and extended networks of people, drive many of us to accept unreasonable restrictions in the guise of safety.

I remember the days after 9-11, in 2001. Americans pulled together in ways they had not since WWII and haven't since. But for a few weeks, at least, we were all one. Behind that feeling of solidarity and togetherness was a Fear of Death: ours, our children's, our friends', our countrymen, and our way of life. We watched death happen in real time on television every day, and then re-watched it over and over again. Then we went to war, mostly to avenge those deaths. At the time of this writing, we're still at war.

Our Fear of Death overtakes us emotionally, and we are led around by that Fear, both consciously and subconsciously, by those who would profit from it. Our Fear of Death compels us to accept new restrictions on our personal freedoms, restrictions we should never allow. To lose one's freedom is tantamount to death, anyway. This Fear has, for millennia, been employed as a tool to manipulate large groups of people to do atrocious things: the Holocaust, Stalin's Purges, the Crusades, Jihads, the Vietnam War, Japanese Internment Camps, the Indian Wars of the 19th century, forced migrations of millions of people following WWI, the list goes on and on, and on.

There's very little point in holding a Fear of Death. Everyone dies; that's just the natural reality. And we shouldn't be overly concerned about *how* we die, or *when*, because there is absolutely *no way* to know either of those two things in advance. They exist in the future, which doesn't exist.

If we're going to fear something, we should rather fear that we will not actually *live*. And if we we walk around afraid of dying then we'll never truly live in the first place. If you aren't actually *living* your life then you're dead already, and there's nothing to fear, because death is already here.

The Fear of Death is Death *Itself*. It is, in fact, the only thing to Fear about dying.

FEAR OF REJECTION

We've all been rejected at one time or another, probably many times. It's a painful experience and one that we all fear.

"What if I try out for the school play, the baseball team, or apply for that job, and I'm rejected?"

It's not a comforting thought. Rejection rocks our self-esteem. The Fear of Rejection could fall under the category of Pain of Outcome, since it's a type of failure, but I think it fits more squarely under Pain of Loss. What we lose when we're rejected is our self-esteem, confidence and, sometimes, our relationships. Rejection is a heavy blow.

Dr. Noah St. John, in *The Book of Afformations©: Discovering the Missing Piece to Abundant Health, Wealth, Love, and Happiness*, argues that the Fear of Rejection is the "most basic human fear." He suggests that this goes back to the earliest human tribal roots, where to be rejected by your tribe meant banishment. This in turn meant that your chances of survival alone in the wild was next to nil.

While I think the Fear of Rejection is a prominent and ancient Fear, and while I think Dr. St. John's book is amazing (one that I strongly suggest reading, and will come back to later in the book when we examine methods to combat Fear) I'm going to respectfully and cordially, disagree that it is the *basic* Fear that drives all the others.

I think the base Fear in the situation that Dr. St. John poses isn't really rejection; it's Death. What does the tribe-member *really* fear? Is it rejection? Being rejected is painful, no doubt about it. We've all felt it many times. But at the base of rejection is what? I think it is what will happen *after* we're kicked out of the tribe, our group, our family, our society: namely, we might die, or at the very least, suffer loads of pain. That might be physical pain but certainly psychological pain, the Pain of Loss.

There's more than one form of loss and rejection, as we'll see. A particularly nasty one is criticism.

FEAR OF CRITICISM

I am the product of a cracked musical note.

I exist here, on planet Earth, because of a missed note on a coronet on a street corner in La Grange, Georgia, in 1917.

One bad note, and the path for my existence, and that of many others, was laid. This is the absolute truth. It is a butterfly effect if ever there was one.

This very book you are reading right now began 100 years ago on a dusty corner in a tiny town in the American South, with a single musical mistake: a cracked E flat.

Lieutenant Bivans cracked a note.

An old tuba player and his musical family heard it.

I was born.

This book was written.

John Bivans was a fresh new officer out of The Salvation Army Training School in New York City. He had been assigned to a remote location for a boy from Brown, Ohio. He was now the officer in charge of a small outpost in La Grange, Georgia, about 20 miles west of Atlanta, a town with dirt streets surrounded by farms. As he did with everything, he threw himself into his work with abandon. His mission was to bring the *Word of God* to the people.

He was standing on a corner downtown — if such a small town could have such a thing — holding an 'open air' meeting, something the Salvation Army used to be famous for, but now rarely do. It was a dying phenomenon when I was a kid in the 70s and 80s, but in 1914, it was still in full force.

"What's an open air meeting?" you ask.

Just what it sounds like. A group of Salvationists — that's what they call themselves — would stroll, or march, out into the middle of town, pick a corner and hold a church meeting right there in public. The institution had deep roots, going back to the early days of the organization in the East End of London, home to cobblestones, brothels, and Jack the Ripper.

La Grange, Georgia, didn't have a Ripper, or cobblestones. But it did have a new movie theater. Of course, the movies were silent in those days. If you wanted a soundtrack you had to hire real, live musicians to play back behind the screen, or in an orchestra pit. That's where the Longino family come in to our little story.

Ansel Longino had four children, all of them musicians like their father. Ansel played the tuba and apportioned the rest of the band to his growing family. Somewhere down the line was his daughter, Willie, a beautiful girl, about 18 years old, who played the coronet, which is basically a mellow sounding trumpet.

The Longinos were walking home that fateful evening from a gig at the theater. They were carrying their instruments in cases, strolling down the dirt streets of their home town, when they heard and saw a young man in uniform playing on his coronet. The sounds of the coronet cut through the street noises. The family paused to listen for a moment. And then it happened.

John Bivans destroyed an E-flat.

Now, many amateur musicians would have stopped playing and slunk off in embarrassment after producing such a note, but not Lt. Bivans. Oh no. He continued unabated, as if nothing had happened.

"Any man brave enough to produce a note *that* bad and continue playing, deserves some help," uttered Daddy Longino.

So the Longino family crossed the street, sat their cases down, opened them up, lifted their brass horns, and joined in with the young officer. By the end of that open air meeting, the Longino family had been recruited as the newest members of the La Grange, Georgia, Salvation Army Band. That was the strength of my grandfather's personality. He was a master recruiter with a magnetic charisma that was hard to resist.

And it was due to that charisma, and to his bravery in the face of criticism, that led to the fateful meeting, and eventual *merging*, of two families—the Bivanses and the Longinos. Just a couple years later, John Bivans and Willie Longino were married and she went off to train to be a Salvation Army officer, too. The two of them became famous throughout the southern United States for starting new Salvation Army churches, but more so for teaching over 1,000 people to play brass instruments, leaving bands in their wake wherever they went.

They also had seven children: six girls, and finally, one boy: Samuel John Bivans, my father.

If it hadn't been for the courage of my grandfather that day in La Grange, Georgia, and his ability to ignore his Fear of Criticism, I would not be here writing this book.

If John Bivans *had* a Fear of Criticism, he plowed right through it, earning him the assistance of one of the great family bands in southern history, a wife, children, and a slew of grand and great grand children. Luckily for me, and you, his coronet playing wasn't as flawless as his courage.

How many opportunities have been missed in history because we, or someone else, gave up for Fear of being criticized?

Criticism, a Road-block, and a Dead Yankee General

Just yesterday evening, I went to pick up Paysh from work. I had had a good day, all in all, and her day had been okay, though her legs were killing her due to a very long country walk we had taken on Sunday. She just wanted to go home, after we went to pick up a prescription from the drug store and something for dinner.

That's where the trouble began.

We had to drive down Robert Street.

Robert Street in West St. Paul is one of the ugliest streets in America. Maybe it's not *the* ugliest, but I'd put it up against most. It's a perfect example of that first ring suburban sprawl that began in the '50s and '60s, and was exacerbated by massive, corporate chain stores in the '70s and '80s. In the process, it fell out of the Tree of Ugly and hit every damned branch on the way down.

For the last year or two, the city of West St. Paul has been reconstructing Robert Street, and they're still at it. It has been a complete cluster-fuck the entire time. I'm surprised that any of the businesses along that road have survived because, for long stretches at a time, you can't drive up or down it. Instead, you have to navigate to the place you need to go, via back streets and side streets, mostly guessing which direction is going to work, *this time*. That's because it changes almost daily. It's like a rat maze where the cheese is constantly moved around and the walls of the maze shift every couple of seconds, just about the time you think you've figured out how to get to the cheddar.

I hate going to West St. Paul.

I don't have anything against the people of the city; I'm sure they're all fine, friendly folk. In fact, I know quite a few people who live there. But that street drives me nuts.

Why am I talking about a street in a chapter on criticism?

Good question.

It's because after we picked up the prescription and dropped off some old clothes at Goodwill, we attempted to drive further up Robert to get to Culver's (a midwestern fast-food joint) to pick up some burgers for dinner. I took a parallel street to reach the cross street, Maria, which is how I've always gone to Culver's. But when we turned down Maria, the intersection was closed. There were orange cones, barrels, and barricades blocking the way. We could not cross through the intersection to the other side where the burgers resided.

I lost my happy helmet.

It was entirely illogical but I lost my composure. I was so tired of dealing with the construction on Robert, and all the constant changes, that I launched into a tirade on how pathetic the construction is in Yankeeland, how moronic the engineers were, the city, the planners, I think I even blamed General Tecumsah Sherman even though he wasn't from Minnesota—just because he was a Yankee.

I immediately turned into the parking lot of Lowe's to turn around and find another cross street to get to Culver's. That's when the criticism began, or at least that's how my ears heard it.

Paysh, trying to help resolve a whirlpool of piss that was already spinning, asked me why I had turned around.

"Because I can't go through the fucking intersection!" I snapped back.

"There's a detour sign pointing to the right." she said.

"Why didn't you tell me that a second ago, before I turned in here?" I was really losing my grip on civility, which only made it worse, of course, because I was *aware* that I was losing it. I really hate to lose control, but losing it I was, despite a part of my brain that was still trying to be logical.

Long story short, we eventually got to our burgers, after several ridiculous detours, which Paysh helped me navigate, while I snapped at her the entire way.

Why did I lose my Happy Helmet?

The best I can figure, is that as soon as my emotions began to spin, my internal critic—the one that blamed road construction on a long-dead Yankee general of the Civil War—flipped a switch and turned on some deep seated *self*-criticism. I'm not sure how that works, but it may be that when we begin to criticize others, our self-criticism follows like night follows day. I suspect that's true. It certainly did in my case. But I didn't feel the criticism as *self-*

directed; I felt it as Paysh-directed. It was coming from *her*, not *me*. At least, that's how I perceived it.

She didn't mean it that way, of course, but in my self-critical mind, and the whirlpool of critical piss that I was experiencing at that moment, I could hear my mother's voice from my childhood, pointing out the things I had forgotten to do, or had not done the way she wanted them done, and I reacted with negative energy.

Where does the Fear of Criticism arise? What is its root?

I think the Fear of Criticism comes, in part, from the Fear of the Pain of Loss. We feel that if we make a mistake that we will lose face in the eyes of our peers, or in the case of Lt. Bivans, in the eyes of the public.

The roots of it stem from negative feedback or criticism that we've received in our life. For me, I guess that comes from my mom. She's not gonna like this little chapter, but I think it's necessary to talk about it.

My mom is a tough critic, something she passed along to me. Now, sometimes a critical eye serves us well. It's served *me* well many times. Finding flaws or things to improve can be a good thing, if not carried too far. It's my ability to look at things with an extremely critical eye that allowed me to examine the topic of Fear and write this book.

But being too critical becomes a detriment. I think we would be better served in life looking for things that *are* working, and scale those up, as opposed to trying to fix everything that *isn't* working. A critical eye can keep you from going down some stupid paths, occasionally. So, for that, I thank my mother (though I traveled many a stupid path despite her best efforts. Those paths were mine, not hers).

No one on Earth is a harsher critic of Steve Bivans, than Steve Bivans himself. The things I say to myself would get someone else a black eye or a broken jaw. And since I haven't punched another person in the face in a very long time, no one talks that kind of crap about me, but *me*. Harsh self-criticism isn't good. I'm working on it, but I have a long way to go.

Perhaps worst of all, if there is too much criticism early in life, one tends to grow up to resent any and all kinds of criticism, even if it's meant to be constructive. I think it also contributes to another related Fear, the Fear of Being Wrong, which of course just means that you're afraid of the criticism that comes with being wrong: criticism from others, but even more painful, *self*-criticism.

Fear of Being Wrong

"If you are afraid of being lonely, don't try to be right." — Jules Renard, French writer, pacifist, and general hard ass

"Being right *ain't the same thing as being* effective." —Steve Bivans, author, troublemaker, and self-quoter

"Mr. Bivans! Why haven't you finished your homework?" inquired Coach Lee, with a heavy dose of irritation.

"Didn't feel like it, or need to," I replied with more than a little surprise and a heavy dose of *hubris*.

In the spring of 1983, I was 16 years old and indestructible. I was also a pretty good student, at least as good as a slack-assed teenage boy can be, I suppose. Mostly I skated through the three years I spent at Walter M. Williams High School. I don't remember doing any homework during those three years, though I'm sure I probably did, once or twice. I relied on my test scores to sail through my adolescent academic experience with a solid B average. But in Coach Lee's geometry class, I had a perfect average: 100 plus.

Geometry was easy peasy for me, especially the way Coach Lee taught it. He approached it from a very logical point of view, which suited my temperament nicely. And Coach Lee didn't grade homework. Yeah, I said it. He didn't grade homework. What a brilliant concept! And since he didn't bother to *grade* it, I didn't bother to *do* it. Sure, I'd do one or two or three problems in class after he assigned them, to make sure I really 'got it,' but that was it; I stopped, closed my book and stared at girls the rest of class, or whispered to my buddies around me.

This was no small thorn in the Coach's side, let me assure you. It wasn't because I didn't do the homework, not really. No, it was because I didn't do the homework, and then aced every test, plus bonus points, every fuckin' week. And this situation was beginning to punch cracks in Coach Lee's **Universal Law of Homework Doing**. Yeah, he had a rule, a law, that he would announce once a week when he went around to see who was actually *doing* their homework.

"I want everyone to take our their notebooks and turn to the homework!" Lee would announce with an air of authority that only a bald-headed, state-championship-tennis coach could muster.

Then he would stroll around the room like the British school master from Pink Floyd's *The Wall*, up and down the aisles, glancing down at my fellow students' scribbles of ink and graphite.

"Tommy, why didn't you finish your homework?"

"Uhhh, I didn't get it?" Tommy would answer.

"That's why you're in the *Slow-Laner* group, son," and he would move on down the line, up and down, until he reached me. He would see that I hadn't done it, and just move on. (*Slow-laners* was Coach Lee's pre-P.C. term for students that weren't smart enough to understand geometry, or anything else).

With that ritual concluded, he would walk to the front of the class, spread his feet shoulder-length apart, put his hands behind his back, throw his shoulders back, and give the following speech with the authority you would expect from a Southern high school coach:

"Ladies and Gentlemen. In this class, unlike most classes, you have the right to *do* or *not* to do your homework. You also have the right to pass this class, or FAIL THIS CLASS!" and then he would move on to the lesson for the day. The implication of this law, of course, was that you either did homework or failed the class. It was a binary law. That's the way coachy math teachers like things: black or white, ones or zeros.

Up to that point, I had received a wide berth during these exhortations, because Coach Lee knew I wasn't doing the homework but had the highest math average in the entire high school. Why did he avoid me? I think he was afraid of jeopardizing his precious *law* if he confronted me on it. But this day was different, for some reason.

Maybe it was because there were more 'non-doers-of-homework' in the room that afternoon? I don't know. Probably. He was probably afraid that I was becoming a *bad influence* on my fellow students, a corrupting force. I've been called that a few times since, go figure. I should put it on my fuckin' business cards:

Steve Bivans, Bad Influence, Corrupting Force, and Stand-Up Philosopher
So that day, when the ominous Coach Lee approached my desk, halfway up the aisle, I was unconcerned, as always.

Why would I be? He'd never commented on my lack of homework doing before; why would today be any different?

I was mistaken.

I had crossed some Rubicon, like Caesar running blindly into the dark. Only Caesar *knew* he'd crossed a forbidden boundary. I had no fuckin' clue. I suppose my own *hubris* had blinded me to the realities of the building tension between teacher and student. Hey, I was 16: pretty much clueless by nature.

"Mr. Bivans, why haven't you finished your homework?"

What the fuck? I thought in my head. *Why is he asking me this, NOW?*

The only thing I could come up with was the truth. I was stunned and unable to come up with a lie that might work, and it wouldn't have anyway. Coach Lee had a very sharp bullshit meter, so I uttered the only thing I could think of: the truth, "Didn't feel like it, or need to."

Something in the distance, in a galaxy far, far away, fell off a shelf. You could almost hear it: a tiny, snapping sound, or crash, like an antique decanter of bourbon or brandy falling off of grandma's shelf, shattering on the floor. Possibly it was a tiny capillary in my teacher's brain?

The classroom went silent. A dropped pin or human hair would have shattered the silence.

Coach Lee had played his hand, and I had countered. The ball was in his court.

There must have been a moment, a split second of doubt that ran through his mind between my return and his volley, where he experienced just the slightest Fear: a Fear that he might just *lose* this match if he didn't walk away. But the time for walking away had past; he had served the challenge. Everyone waited with bated breath to see if his *backhand* was as good as his serve, or if their fellow student had the footwork and backspin to sneak a return into the corner.

"Mr. Bivans," Coach Lee countered, "I want you to take your homework to the back of the class. I want you to complete every assigned problem. And for every one you get wrong, I'm going to subtract a point from your next test."

Damn!

It was a pretty strong backhand, for sure.

There could be no mistaking what was going on at this point. Coach Lee was afraid. He was afraid of being wrong. His ***Universal Law of Homework Doing*** was under challenge, and he was having none of it. He was drawing a line in the sand, and daring me to cross it.

"Yes sir," I replied, with no sound of Fear in my voice. I stood up, grabbed my notebook and textbook, confidently strode to the back of the room, and sat down at the *trouble-maker's desk* —you know, the one where old school teachers sent the rabble-rousers: a *time out* desk it might be called, these days.

I went to work.

The room returned their gaze to the Coach, who tried to focus on teaching the day's lesson, feigning to ignore the fact that his law, and reputation for being right, were hanging in the balance. Except for the sound of the Coach's voice booming off the walls, there was no other sound in the room. Everyone was waiting to see the outcome of this challenge.

After about 15 minutes, Coach Lee—impatient for the outcome of the game—called 'time up.'

"Mr. Bivans." all sound in the room ceased, again.

"Yes?" I looked up from my work. I didn't raise my head, only my eyes, as if to look through my eyebrows.

"Are you about finished back there?" the Coach inquired.

"I have a couple problems left to solve."

"Good enough." he replied, "Bring it up here."

If it had been quiet in the room before, the silence deepened in the next few moments. I mean, it was like we had found Absolute Zero, and the vibration of every atom, electron, and quark had ceased. The only sound was the sound of my feet on the floor as I strode to the front of the room. I think my fellow students actually froze in place.

This was an historic moment, and everyone in the class knew it, including the Coach.

I knew if there was *anything* remotely out of place in any of my answers, he was *not* going to give me the benefit of the doubt: no way in *hell* was he going to do *that*. I had to be perfect, or fail. There was no middle ground in this game: no tie, no kissing your sister. It was win, or fuckin' lose.

I handed my notebook to Coach Lee.

The Coach reached back behind him and lifted his textbook.

He turned to the answer key.

Coach looked at my first answer, then at the key.

He moved to the next answer, then back to his book.

Over and over again, he scanned: answer, key, answer, key, answer, key.

This took one thousand years, if it took a minute.

The silence deepened in anticipation of the verdict. It felt as if the gravity in the room had increased, like suddenly moving from Earth to Jupiter. There was a palpable tension, a mammoth suspense in the air. Time itself had been suspended.

The clock stopped.

The sun itself paused in the heavens, and the Earth refused to spin on its axis, for only a second, but it might as well have been a year.

"They're all correct," the Coach uttered.

He did so, not in the voice of defeat; that was never gonna happen with Coach Lee. He spoke with resolution, not with resignation. I think, also, there was just a *hint* of pride in that voice: pride in the accomplishment of a student, his student. But he knew as well as everyone else in the room, that the Rubicon had been crossed, and that the rules were now changed.

The Universe had altered itself.

The next week, Coach Lee began his homework checking speech, with the following announcement:

"Ladies and Gentlemen. In this class, unlike most classes, you have the right to *do* or *not* do your homework. *IN MOST CASES*, if you choose the latter, you will FAIL THIS CLASS!" and glanced at me while he said it.

A Deadly Fruit

One of the deadliest fears of all is the Fear of Being Wrong.

I say deadly, not because it always leads to death — nothing died in my 10th grade geometry class with the exception of a small portion of Coach Lee's *hubris* — but because the *potential* for massive destruction and death is always there.

This is the Fear that has driven friends to part, spouses to attack, neighbors to murder, and entire nations to war.

It creates conflict over ideologies, religions, and national identities. It brings into focus the false sense of *otherness*, especially other people, and creates a harsh sense of Us versus Them. It is one of the roots of nationalism, bigotry, racism, and all forms of intolerance.

When it takes control of the mind, it entrenches it behind metaphorical walls and throws up boundaries: psychological, physical, and imagined. It is the driving force behind the imaginary political boundaries of the world. We have divided up the planet with these imaginations and given them symbols: flags, statues, slogans, and anthems. All of this reinforces the Fear of the Other.

The Fear of Being Wrong leads to intransigence, pig-headedness, closed-mindedness, defensiveness, anger, conflict, and war. It is the force that drove the Nazi Party to gas and incinerate six million Jews and another five million souls that didn't fit their model of being *right*, i.e., Arian. It was the driving force behind Stalin's Purges, which left over 20 million Russians buried in mass graves all over Eastern Europe and Western Asia. It is the Fear that led the U.S. into Korea and Vietnam, convinced that their way was *right* and that communism was *wrong*.

It creates threats out of thin air. If I am *right* and you are *wrong*, then you instantly become a potential, if not real, enemy. I must protect myself and my friends, family, and nation against your threat.

What is *right*?

What is *wrong*?

If you examine the discussion of these two questions throughout the history of philosophy, you will find no real consensus. The closest thing to such a consensus is that it's wrong to cause harm to someone else. One might argue that there's a consensus on that point. But is there a single group of people on Earth living by that philosophy?

If the so-called, *free-est* nation on Earth, the United States, can't follow it, then who can? Who will?

The U.S. has been in so many wars—and is still embroiled in a protracted one as I write this—that it long ago gave up any right whatsoever to argue that others shouldn't also start and engage in war, or any other kind of oppression. Our record on oppressing other people is appalling; just examine what we did to the native population within our own borders. And that's only the beginning.

The Fear of Being Wrong has tainted all borders, all nations, every religion (even Buddhism), and every ideology. Even science isn't clean on this one. In fact, it might be one of the most egregious ideologies around. While most scientists will argue that science isn't an ideology, and maybe in theory they're right, it certainly has underlying metaphysical assumptions about how the Universe works, and those are mostly *unexamined* assumptions. Those assumptions lead many scientists to defend academic positions long after it is prudent to do so and long after the facts and evidence suggest that they should.

Of course, scientists aren't alone; this is a problem for the entire species. *Homo sapiens* love to be right, and are deathly afraid of being wrong. We fuckin' hate it. And I'm here to tell you, yours truly is guilty as well, maybe more so than most people.

What Drives This Fear?

I think there are at least two things behind the Fear of Being Wrong.

One, if we have to admit that something we believed is wrong, we take a massive hit to our self-esteem. And this is a big deal. We spend all of our lives trying to protect what little self-esteem we have. If we have to admit being wrong about something important, especially something that we have long believed to be true, it knocks us on our ass for awhile, if not permanently.

This makes us very defensive of our ideas and ideals. We protect them with vehemence and anger. We physically cross our arms in defensiveness during an argument, we back up, we withdraw, and we throw up those metaphorical walls to protect ourselves from the truth, or the *lie* that someone else is attacking us with.

We do all this because of the second thing behind the Fear of Being Wrong: we think that *what we believe* is *who we are*.

WHO ARE WE? FEAR OF THE LOSS OF IDENTITY

Who Are We?

Humans have a curious way of defining themselves. I should say that we have *many* curious ways of doing it. Here's an exercise that's kind of fun.

Ask yourself, "Self, how many of you *are* there?"

I'm not suggesting that you have multiple personality disorder, though in a way, you do. So do I. When I asked myself that question some months ago, I got enough answers to fill up at least one page on a legal pad.

How many Steve Bivanses are there? A lot of them.

I am,

- A Southerner
- a writer
- a coach
- a strategic advisor
- an historian
- a farmers market manager
- a food activist
- a cat lover
- a dad
- a boyfriend
- a sword swinger
- an axe thrower
- a BBQ master
- a soup maker
- Mr. Mom
- a chauffeur
- a graduate student
- and a bunch more things

You can see that we can all define ourselves in so many ways, because we do so many things. But are these who we *are*? That's a philosophical question that we don't have time to go into in this book. But it's worth considering for a second just how many labels we put on ourselves and that doesn't include those we receive from others. These are *hats* we wear, depending on the situation. We change them constantly.

But we are much slower to change our *beliefs*, something *else* we often use to define ourselves: I'm a Christian, a Muslim, a Jew, a Buddhist, a Democrat, a Republican, and on and on. While these are all just labels, most of us adopt them and redefine what they mean, to us. Then we put a lot of faith and belief into them. The word belief implies, within its definition, that there is the slightest uncertainty, because it doesn't require proof or hard evidence. We *accept* an idea as true, but somewhere deep in our minds is a Fear that we might just be *wrong*. And we feel we have to defend that belief, sometimes all the way to violence, war, and death.

Why do we do this?

I think it's because we have an internal mechanism that equates *who we are* with *what we currently believe*. Our beliefs, in other words, aren't just things we *have* or that we *hold on to*, they come to define our very *being*, our sense of self. We *are* what we *believe* about the world, about the origins of all things, about our relationships, about ourselves, about everything. We are seriously attached to our beliefs. They have become *things*; they have become *us*. We are our beliefs, and our beliefs are us. We have bound up our very *identity* within them. Coach Lee *identified* with his Universal Law of Homework-Doing, *"If you don't do your homework, you will fail this class!"* He took a major hit of self-identity when he found out it wasn't a law, after all.

I am what I believe.

That's a very powerful statement. And most of us never really think about it, about how our beliefs shape our very existence, our identity, our place in the cosmos and the history of the world. Beliefs aren't just ideas; they have become things, they have become us. They are nouns, in other words. And nouns are very powerful things; they are concrete, factual, *real*.

From Belief to Believing?

But what if we turned beliefs into verbs? Make them more transient, fluid, ever-changing? What if, instead of *having* these things, these nouns called *beliefs*, we instead experienced them as verbs? Instead of having beliefs, we could just experience *believing*. It's a very small change in our way of thinking, but with massive ramifications.

If, in a conversation, you say that you know the distance from the Earth to the Sun is 93.whatever-million-miles, and I come back with "That's a useable theory for most predictions," we might continue to have a civil discussion, whereas if I say, "That's complete bullshit," you might punch me in the face, and then I'd have to kick your ass, your family would come after me, and soon there'd be a world war with button pushing and mushroom clouds popping up all over the planet.

Okay, that was an exaggeration, maybe, but you get the point. If I don't hold onto my Fear of Being Wrong, or certainty of being right—the distance between the Earth and the Sun is actually zero —then I could ask you some questions about your theory, as long as you aren't entrenched in the idea that it's 93.whatever-million-miles away. If you don't feel threatened, if you're just currently *believing* about the distance from the Earth to the Sun, instead of feeling like your *belief* and sense of *self* is in danger, then a conversation can happen, instead of an argument and full-on nuclear war.

The best way to combat the Fear of Being Wrong is to assume that most of the time the things we think are solid, factual, or *right* are, in fact, *theories*. Or maybe I should say they are in *theory* theories. Most of what we think is solid, even the chair you sit upon, isn't solid at all. And the reason the Sun isn't 93-whatever-million-miles away is due to two reasons.

One, the Earth's orbit is elliptical, not circular, so the distance changes constantly. It's never a set distance; it fluctuates based on what day, hour, minute, second, millisecond, microsecond we're talking about.

Two, our planet isn't solid, or uniform. Where would we hold the end of the tape measure? On the top of Mt. Everest, or the bottom of the Marianas Trench out in the Pacific Ocean? Big difference.

The Sun isn't solid, either, even less so than the Earth. It isn't a big, shiny rubber ball out in space. It doesn't have a surface on which to place our tape measure to measure the distance between it and our blue planet. Where would we hold the tape measure on the Sun? At the core? But where is the edge of the sun? Is it the tip of the longest solar flare? Good luck measuring that!

Maybe it's the furthest reaches of the Sun's light? Now there is the real answer. That light is in one instant, *wave*, and in another instant, *particle*, so not only does the light—the waves of the Sun—reach us here on Earth, but also its particles. Ergo, the distance from the Sun to the Earth, is actually zero. Think about it for a while. It might just blow your mind and occasion you to question everything else you think you know, including the belief that you have no control over your life.

LOSS OF STATUS: LONE TREE? OR UNIVERSAL FOREST?

One belief that most of us feel is that we are alone in the world.

That doesn't mean that we don't have friends, or family, or we're not part of larger communities. What it means is that, down deep, we all feel as if we are a tiny cog in a vast machine: the Universe. This belief, if carried too far, can result in an individual adopting the status of victim.

Victim Status: What's the Benefit?

It's easy, especially when things in life haven't turned out the way we wanted, to think that the world is against us, that the gods have forsaken us. Even the progenitor of Christianity, Jesus, got to that point, "Father, why has't thou forsaken me?" If he could reach that point, how easy and how normal can it be for us to reach that point, as well?

It is this inner feeling of disconnectedness that can lead us to feel like victims, as if we have no power over our lives. I've been there. It's not a place anyone ever *wants* to be. But sometimes, once we're in it, we get kind of comfortable in our misery, and that's just messed up.

Why would anyone claim victim status?

One of the things that I've learned in the last year or so is that if we have a core negative belief—*I'm not enough, I'm doomed, I'm lazy, I'm a victim of Fate*—it's because that status is benefitting us in some way, or we think it is. Down deep it might actually be killing us, because it prevents us from reaching the very success that we want in life. But on some level, in our subconscious at least, there has to be a belief that this victim status is serving us; otherwise, our mind would not permit it. Our mind always does exactly what it *thinks* we want. *Our mind does what it thinks we want it to do.*

We tell it what we want all the time. This is something that therapist, Marisa Peer, emphasizes. We are constantly giving our mind instructions. The problem is, that most of them are negative instructions. And if we think we will get something out of being a victim, then we subconsciously tell our minds that we *are* victims.

What is the benefit of being a victim?

Sympathy, for one. If we can convince others that we are simply victims of circumstances they will feel sorry for us, pay attention to us, maybe do things for us. Most of this runs automatically in our subconscious.

The main benefit of a victim status is that it allows us to shift responsibility away from ourselves onto others, or onto the gods, or the Universe, or the government, or global capitalism. Sometimes all of these are guilty of gross injustice, malice, corruption, greed, even war and murder. There *are* real victims in the world, and most of us have been one at some time or another in our lives. No doubt about it.

You're a Victim. So What?

But even if you *are* a victim, so what?

Sorry if I sound harsh, but this is a reality that we must face if we want to be anything *but* a victim the rest of our lives. Even if we are a genuine and true victim, what good does it do us to hang onto that status? Other than the weak reasons I gave above—sympathy and avoidance of responsibility—why hold on to it? There is no reason. Being a victim in your own mind will never turn you into a success. NEVER. If you think it will, you got another *think* comin'. It will not.

If you want to keep it in a drawer somewhere as a badge, or scar, fine; do it. You can pull it out years from now when you're giving your TED Talk, or running for President, or as your opening speech to your corporation as CEO. You can talk about how the world tried to keep you down but you kicked its ass anyway. That's the only decent use of victim status. Otherwise, drop it.

In the end, the world doesn't care if you're a victim. Yeah, you might get some sympathy, even from me, and that's okay. But that sympathy ain't gonna make you a success.

Sympathy doesn't equal Success. It never has and it never will. Cut ties with that part of your identity.

Question Everything

Don't be so quick to believe things. Question the fuck out of them. Question EVERYTHING, especially your own beliefs, including the beliefs about *who you are*. Don't become a rock. Rocks aren't solid either, if you look close enough. Stop being solid. And stop being a victim. Be more fluid with your beliefs and your sense of self. If you do, then you won't be inclined to defend what you think is right, and you can say goodbye to the Fear of Being Wrong.

Many times, our victim status is attached to the things we *lack* in life: money, love, status, appreciation. So let's take a close look at one of the biggest, nastiest fruits on the Tree of Fear: the Fear of Scarcity.

Fear of Scarcity

One of the so-called, *driving forces* of the world's problems is the idea that all of the Earth's resources are scarce: water, food, land, and money. This Fear of Scarcity has, and is, leading the planet into disaster after disaster. It's one of the driving forces behind every war in history, and is behind our insatiable drive to take more and more from our environment, damn the consequences. In the wake of this Fear is pollution, extinction of species, and a ravaged climate.

A Scarcity mentality drives greed, a desire for more and more money, not only by the richest of the rich, but by the rest of us who want a piece of that pie. In our minds, everything is scarce, so we better get it now before it's all gone. But it's the very mentality that things are scarce that makes them so. Without our rabid Fear of Scarcity, we could find ways to more equitably *use* the abundant resources that do exist on our planet. Instead of killing each other over the possession of them, we could work together to find ways to share them and even *increase* them.

Money and Scarcity: the Law of Attraction

I hear a lot these days about the idea that money is an energy force that flows freely, or can flow freely, through the world. Much of this talk comes in the context of the idea of the Law of Attraction.

The Law of Attraction, as I understand it, essentially states that we attract to us those things to which we are in alignment.

I know all that sounds very New Age-y, *Woo Woo*, and mystical. And trust me, I'm really *not* into the *Woo Woo*. But I'm not sure it has to be *Woo Woo-ey*. There's some pretty sound logic behind the idea, even if the scientific community hasn't given it much credit or examined it closely.

Let's take money, for instance. Many of us have a fear of not having enough money to pay our bills, put food on the table, and live a life that is free from worry. I know it's always been a huge worry for me, and I know I'm not alone.

The Law of Attraction would say that it is the very Fear of Scarcity that creates the lack of money in the first place. The Fear that we have manifests itself in the very thing that we *don't* want: scarcity. Think about it this way. How many times have you been afraid that something bad was going to happen? So much so, that you prepared for this disaster, had nightmares about it, and worried about it during the day, every day, and then it happened? Maybe not exactly as you had imagined it, but in a similar way? We tend to put ourselves *into* the very situations that we want to avoid, by focusing on them constantly. That's what the Law of Attraction is all about. It's not mystical; it's very practical and logical.

I think it's easier to see when we talk about relationships. Imagine a person who is insanely jealous. Someone so worried that their significant other will cheat on them or find someone else, that they are constantly interrogating their mate about where they've been, what they've been doing, and who they've been with. Can you see what direction this relationship is headed? Who is manifesting that direction: the significant other or the jealous mate? What do you think is going to happen in this example? There are infinite outcomes, but it's likely that the relationship will fail — and in epic style — maybe with flames and explosions, like a Tarentino film.

The Fear of Loss will always manifest itself in loss. It will never, ever manifest itself in gain. If you fear losing something, you will lose something, and probably the very thing you most fear to lose. This happens so often that we don't need scientific data to support it; it's just plain logical.

Why would that same logic not apply to everything, even money?

I would argue that it does. If you have a Fear of Scarcity built up around money, which I have always had, then you may work your ass off for years, even decades, and still have no money in your bank account. You may *survive* on a shoestring—I have—but you will not *thrive* and build wealth, at least not of the monetary kind. It is the very mentality of Scarcity that manifests this situation. It is probably at the root of poverty, but the idea can be taken too far.

Is it the Poor's Fault that They're Poor?

One of the things that I resist, when it comes to the Law of Attraction, is the tendency of some proponents to blame the poor for being poor, with the logical fallacy that *"If you are poor, you must have caused that by having a scarcity mentality about money."* Ergo, if they simply removed that mentality and began believing in abundance, they'd be rich.

There are a couple of problems with that theory. One is that it disregards the influence of outside forces when it comes to poverty. Poverty is a man-made problem, not a natural one. But it is not all created from within the individual human mind. Much of it is imposed upon large groups of people due to the Fears that other people have, namely, the Fear of the Other—in the case of race, religion, culture—and the Fear of Scarcity—in the mindsets of some of the world's richest people.

Yes, I said it. Even people *with money* can be living with a Fear of Scarcity. They are so afraid that they'll never have *enough* of whatever it is they want—which appears to be everything on Earth —that they grasp, steal, and exploit their way to the top of the money heap.

Let me be perfectly clear about something. I am *not* saying that *all* rich people are evil, or living in a scarcity mindset. I would not make such a broad judgement. But many wealthy people are deathly afraid of losing their wealth and do everything in their power to hold onto it, horde it, and increase it at any cost. This is true especially among the richest of the world.

"But how can they attract so much wealth, if they have a Fear of Scarcity?"

This is a very good question, and one that brings me to the second thing I resist when it comes to the Law of Attraction.

Attraction vs Extraction

There seems to be a counter theory in the Attraction belief community, that if one is poor because of the Law of Attraction, then if one is rich, it is because that person has aligned themselves in an open way to money and wealth, and therefore, are *worthy* of that wealth. But money doesn't only come to people via attraction. We know this is true.

Money also comes to people via *extraction*: murder, rape, and theft, by exploiting one's workers, paying less than livable wages, skimping on healthcare for one's employees, making shoddy products to push off on the public to maximize profits; the list goes on. There are endless ways to accrue a fortune, all while in the scarcity mindset.

But the question remains whether these *extractors* can hold *onto* that wealth. It certainly seems that they can, or do, in many cases. So where does that leave the Law of Attraction?

If some people manage to extract, or accrue, so much money by coercive means, what does that mean for our Law of Attraction? Will they be able to hold onto it? If they do, at least in their lifetime, will they suffer other forms of scarcity? I would argue that they do.

The Karma of Greed?

Two of the leaders in the field of positive psychology (as opposed to clinical), Jim Loehr and Martin Seligman, point to studies that demonstrate that after a person accumulates a certain level of wealth, further accumulation has an inverse effect on their happiness and general well-being. It seems that if you extract wealth well beyond what you actually need, it turns on you. The more you have, the less happiness it brings.

This has been questioned, of course, by proponents of the Law of Attraction who argue that there *is* no scarcity and, therefore, a person can accumulate as much wealth as they desire. I don't want to go too far down this rabbit hole, so let's just say that while the statistics strongly suggest that over-accumulation of wealth leads to diminishing returns in happiness and well-being, the numbers are only statistical. And as the great Mark Twain once said, "There are lies, damned lies, and statistics."

Statistics are great for seeing larger trends, but they suck at predicting how individuals will react, or act, in any given situation. For instance, the average lifespan of an American male is 78.7 years. This tells us a lot about the population of men in America. But it doesn't tell us shit about Joe Blow next door, or about when *we* will die. Many men live to be in their 90s, some to 100. Some die in their 30s and 40s. And in the same way, statistics about how wealth accumulation affects our happiness and well-being can be taken with a grain of salt when it comes to the individual.

That being said, the Law of Attraction applies to more things than wealth and money. If an individual goes around extracting from his neighbors, simply to accumulate things for himself, he is in Fear of Scarcity, and he will suffer scarcity in one way or another. Most likely, he'll lose the very things he is extracting. If not, then he will lose something else that he values. One cannot cheat the Law of Attraction any more than Little Red Riding Hood could escape the big bad wolf.

BASKET FULL OF SCARCITY: BIG BAD WOLVES OF DEBT

What's the biggest success blocker in your life? Mine, I think, is the Fear of the wolves outside the door, in the Forest, around the corner, sneaking up behind me, eying the few remaining fruits in my basket.

The Big Bad Wolves

Let me explain.

I—like many people these days—am plagued by financial debt. Thanks to my lack of success in the sphere of money and many adult years in college and graduate school, I have managed to chalk up a lot of debts. And my income won't touch them, not at present anyway.

Those debts—plus the ordinary everyday bills and debt that

we all face—are the *wolves* of which I speak. Some days, when I'm feeling confident in my abilities, or I have enough money in the pocket to at least buy lunch and put some gas in the tank, I don't hear them howling in the Forest.

They are *at bay*, for the moment. I can forget about them for a while.

But they're always out there, and all it takes to get them howling in my ear is the slightest rustle of wind in the trees: a letter from a debt collector, a word from a passing stranger about money troubles, anything related to debt and money. They are lurking behind every tree.

Thanks to my good friend, Greg Dickson, who is a coach and master of what he calls the Emotional Release Approach, I have put most of my angst toward money itself, to rest. I don't think of money as an evil entity anymore. But the lack of money coming *in* creates a circular problem, thanks to the Law of Attraction we were just discussing.

Of course, writing this section will probably bring me *more* lack of money, but I'm gonna write it anyway, because I hope to write myself *out* of that story and into a new one. Also, I hope that by sharing my story it will help *you* to get through the dark Forest and avoid the big bad wolves.

How Do the Wolves of Debt Become a Success Blocker?

There are at least a couple of ways that my fear of debt hinders my success.

One, they create a negative attraction loop, by focusing my mind upon what I *don't have*, instead of allowing me to focus on the process of doing what I do, which will eventually bring me success.

Two, the Fear of the Wolves of Debt creates a recurring brain-spin, what I call my *Whirlpool of Piss* surrounding the very *idea* of success.

How?

When the howling begins, it becomes a massive distraction from my work. I know I can't pay those debts off, and in order for that to *ever* happen, I'll have to be very successful. A little bit of success won't cut it. It's like Tom Petty once sang, "Sometimes I feel, if I don't win, How'm I gonna break even?" I've had that feeling for decades.

Once you've managed to get into a big hole, all you see are the sides of the hole. It's almost impossible to see the sun, except for certain times of the year when it passes directly overhead. And while that view slowly expands as you claw your way up the sides, it doesn't really open up until you're near the top. It's almost like being Grandma in the belly of the Wolf before the heroic woodsman hacks her out of there.

If you're deep in the Forest of Goldilocks, Red-Riding Hood, and Hansel n Gretel, it's hard to see anything but dark, foreboding trees, or hear anything but the howling of wolves, growling of bears, and cackling of witches.

Some days you just can't find the path through the forest, so you stop dead in your tracks, wondering which way to turn next. And then you hear the wolves again.

I don't spend too many days in that Forest. But there are still days when I find myself suddenly surrounded by trees and hearing nothing but wolves. And that is neither enjoyable, nor productive. I get very little done when I'm dodging wolves, and inactivity only increases their number and ferocity.

Inaction and Scarcity: Feeding the Wolves of Debt

I can't kill or elude wolves if I'm sitting still in their Forest. They will eat me alive if I don't keep moving. Winston Churchill once said, "When you're walking through Hell, just keep walking," Can there be better advice?

Here's a lesson for you.

I almost cut this section from the book.

Yep, I didn't think it really fit in anywhere, until today — November 7th, 2016 — when the wolves jumped me in the Forest, again. I was getting on track with the book, nearing the finish, when I suddenly became aware that the basket I was carrying was full of *not-a-whole-fuckin-lot*. It was *full* of scarcity. My basket — my bank account — was empty again. And I heard the howling from around the bend in the Forest path.

Grandma ain't gonna get lunch, today.

And I froze in my tracks.

I got up at 1:50 in the morning with a *Whirlpool of Piss* swirling in my head. Most people refer to it as *brain spin*, or *Monkey Brain*. I also call it my Waring Blender of Dog Shit n Crackers. Not a good recipe for a smoothie, if you know what I mean. And this morning it was howling and spinning with a vengeance. So, I got up, put on my jammy pants, and went downstairs to sit in my overstuffed chair in the office, and brood.

I brooded for hours.

I'm fuckin' broke.

There's nothing to cook for breakfast.

How am I gonna pay all the bills this month?

Where the fuck is the money gonna come from? You get the gist.

And the feeling persisted, all morning, even after taking a two hour nap with Bubble the Dog and Punkin' Kitty. If *that* doesn't cure me, pretty much nothing does.

But then I took a shower, and in the shower—what *is it* with taking showers?—I came to a realization that I was once again being chased by wolves in the Forest, and that I should put this section back in the book. So my Fear of the wolves—the very thing that had stopped me in my tracks—became the motivation to get moving again!

So you can thank the Wolves of Debt that they were included in this book. While in that hot shower, I realized something important. If *I* have such Fears, you might also have them. And if I could figure out how to get moving again, it might encourage *you* to keep moving through the Forest. Don't stop, Miss Hood, Miss Goldilocks, or Mr. Hansel. If you do, the wolves will catch up, and that ain't *ever* good.

If you find yourself in a dark wood and hear the Wolves a howlin', take heart that you've been through Forests before, and survived. They won't kill you as long as you don't stop. Keep walking my friend. Do *something* positive, however small it may be. Pay one bill, a small one. Gaze at one beautiful flower outside your window. Pet your dog or cat—if they'll let you (Squishy Kitty is actually sleeping next to me on my desk). Hug your wife, husband, children, and take a deep breath.

You're gonna be okay.

Fear only brings us more of what we don't want.

For now, we're going to leap like a squirrel from the Widow-Maker branch of Loss to the most twisted branch on the Tree: the Fear of the Pain of Process.

Climbing a Crooked Branch: Change and the Fear of Pain of Process

Of the three major branches on the Tree of Fear, I think the one most overlooked is the crooked branch of the Fear of the Pain of Process. I think this is because most of us don't think of process as something we 'Fear,' just something that we don't *like*. But if you don't like something, especially if you *really* don't like it, to the point of *not doing it*, then there is definitely Fear involved.

The Fear of Process is a very subtle one, and it has two particularly elusive fruits: the Fear of Chaos and the Fear of Starting. Both tend to stop us in our tracks from achieving many of the goals we set for ourselves.

Once we begin to make plans for the future, we begin to worry about the uncomfortable nature of change. We don't like change and the thought of it, more often than not, occasions Fear.

We are actually very conservative when it comes to the range of experiences we incorporate into our lives. Think of the trepidation you feel when starting any new venture, like a new job, for instance. Remember the first day on your current job? What was that like? How did those feelings manifest themselves physically and mentally? Bet they were very much like encountering snakes or bears.

You see, once Fear kicks in, it always feels the same, because all fears, whether they originate in our *Homo sapiens* Brain, our Monkey Brain, or in our Lizard Brain, are experienced in the Land of the Lizard. All Fear is *felt* in the Lizard Bran. They may originate in our frontal lobe, but they don't stay there. The Lizard Brain doesn't distinguish between lions and your new boss or bears and the imaginary scenarios that you have conjured up about your first day at work. To the Lizard, it's all life and death.

The Fear of the Pain of Process is most acute when we attempt, or want to attempt, something new: change careers, stop smoking, get in better shape, or reach out to our neighbor with the annoying dog. This Fear can stop us dead in our tracks.

What we fear is the discomfort or hassle of going through the process of change. *"I'll have to learn new skills for that job,"* or *"I don't know how to run a business,"* or *"I'll have to get up earlier every morning to write that book,"* or *"I'll have to get new running shoes if I start jogging every day,"* or *"I'll have the shakes and cravings if I stop smoking."*

There are many steps to any goal that we might have in life, and they aren't all easy ones. When we begin the journey toward our goals we naturally have some trepidation about all of those steps.

Change, by its very nature, is uncomfortable. And by *our* very nature, we love the familiar. Familiar things aren't a threat to us, or at least we don't perceive them to be. Sometimes the familiar is dangerous as hell. If you grew up in an abusive family, you might come to think of such a home as *normal*, and subconsciously seek out situations later in life that replicate what was *familiar* to you in childhood. This is one of the things that make abuse such a difficult cycle to break.

But even if the familiar things in our life aren't dangerous, they don't help us to grow, to become all we can be. Sure, sitting in my favorite chair is very comfortable, but what will I learn from it? Will it make me a better person? Will I improve my health, my happiness, or my wealth by sitting here?

If you're reading this book in your favorite chair, just maybe! But if you're just sitting there eating bowls of ice cream, maybe not. Trust me, I've eaten a shit-ton of ice cream in my favorite chair, and as enjoyable as it was, I haven't learned much from the experience, except perhaps, that my jeans keep shrinking.

Change is challenging and not at all comfortable. But people make changes all the time. Do you have children? Now *there's* a change! It's difficult to think of a bigger one, quite frankly. Have you ever changed jobs by choice? Were you fired? That's another big change. The first one is easier to deal with, in some ways, since it was your choice to change but that doesn't mean it's really easy. Sometimes being fired is easier. You don't have to make the choice! It's been made *for you*.

I've been there, for sure. I've been fired a few times in my life. It sucks ass, but at the same time, it's kind of liberating. It pushes you out the door and opens up new opportunities. Of course, it can also leave you homeless and hungry.

Let's climb the crooked branch of Process and take a look at the fruits that grow upon it: the Fears of Chaos, of Missing Out, and of Starting.

Fear of Chaos

I was going to drown.

Another dark wave washed over my head.

All I could taste was salt.

Fuck! I'm gonna fuckin' drown!

In 1986, I was 20 years old. My younger brother, Dave, was in high school. At the time, we lived in New Bern, North Carolina, about a 45 minute drive from the coast. Every Memorial Day weekend, New Bern High School juniors and seniors had a tradition of racing off to the beach to party. Dave was no different, so we packed up our coolers, bodyboards, and bags of chips and headed for the beach.

I won't go into all the details of what happened that first evening. Suffice it to say that we were *impaired* later that night when Dave and I decided to go swimming in the ocean, which was right outside the door of the house that he and his friends had rented for the weekend.

The water was dark and warm. There was a mild surf, not really big enough for bodyboarding, so we just went in to swim.

Minutes later, we were in the jaws of a riptide.

If you don't live near the ocean, you might not be acquainted with this natural phenomenon, so I'll give you a brief explanation.

A riptide occurs when the current of the beach shifts so that it develops an area of stiff, outward current moving away from the beach and out to sea. It can be extremely strong. Attempting to swim against it is suicidal. Riptides claim lives all the time, on beaches around the world. In 2015, in the U.S. alone, 42 people lost their lives to this phenomenon.

Dave and I found ourselves caught in a very strong riptide pulling us away from the beach.

Both of us were born and raised near the water. We were excellent swimmers. In fact, Dave was a certified lifeguard and avid surfer. But try as we might, we could not swim in to shore. The harder we swam, the further out we went. The tide was winning and we were losing energy, fast. The Fear of Death was running through our veins.

Luckily for Dave and I, our good friend, Jimmy, was on shore. He was the only person on the beach. Swimming in the ocean at night isn't the smartest thing to do in the best conditions, but especially so, if no one else is on shore.

Jimmy had noticed that we were struggling to come back in and we yelled to him that we needed help. He snapped into action, grabbed his surfboard from the sand, and dove into the dark ocean to swim out to us. When he finally reached us, Dave and I were all but spent and probably wouldn't have lasted much longer. We gripped ahold of Jimmy's surfboard and started sucking air.

Jimmy then instructed us to do something that both of us already knew — but were unable to remember in our current state — that the only way to escape a riptide is to swim perpendicular to it, at a 90 degree angle, until you get outside of it. Then you can turn toward shore and use the natural current, coming in, to bring you back.

Duh.

I say, duh, but it's not that intuitive, and every year people drown because they don't know this trick, or like Dave and I, are unable to remember it when they need it most.

We all made it back to shore that night, but Dave and I were completely spent of all energy. Were it not for the heroic act of our friend we would both have drowned that night and become a statistic. I would not be here writing this book or telling this story.

Why am I talking about riptides? Because they represent a natural manifestation of *chaos*, and when we try to resist chaos, bad things happen.

Swimming Against Riptides: the Fear of Chaos and Your Imminent Drowning

Have you ever been trying to focus on accomplishing a particular task, but couldn't keep your mind on it?

What distracted you?

For me, it's usually all of the other things I know I need to do that continuously draw my attention away from what I need to do most. I recently read Gary Keller's book, *The One Thing*, in which he dealt with this very phenomenon. He argued, and I agree completely, that most of the time it is our Fear of Chaos that pulls us away from the task at hand to our To Do List.

More often than not, the *to do* list doesn't exist; all those things are just floating around in our brain, clouding up our thinking and screwing up the thing we need to do most with thoughts of the laundry, or dog washing, or mowing the lawn, or picking up the kids from school, or a hundred thousand other tasks that have to be done. We may need to do them, it's true, but most of these tasks aren't really that crucial if we consider them in the grand scheme of things.

The fact that we haven't taken the time to write them down makes them even more distracting, because they are in our head, where we worry that we'll forget them.

Why Do We Fear Chaos?

I think we fear chaos because it represents the ultimate loss of control. We love to feel in control of every situation and we crave order. As a species, we have developed an inner desire for control over our environment and, to a large extent, we have achieved much in that direction. But control is always an illusion. In fact, we have no control over anything, with the possible exception of our own thoughts, but who really has control over those? I certainly do not.

It is the illusion that we *can* control our environment, our friends, our family, every situation, that leads us to fear chaos. This is unfortunate, because chaos rules. Just look around you now. Put down the book for a minute and look around you.

Do you really have control over what's happening?

Is everything in perfect order in your room or outdoor space where you're sitting reading this book? Is it really? If you think so —maybe you're extremely tidy—look closer. Do you see a speck of dust anywhere? A cat hair or dog hair? My house is covered in both, all the time.

There is no such thing as clean. There is no perfection, other than the perfection of chaos itself. The Fear of Chaos is really the love of *perfect order*, the elusive *perfection*. The problem is that perfection doesn't exist. It is an illusion, just like the control it would take to make it a reality. We control nothing. We can certainly *influence* everything around us. But we can never control them, anymore than you can swim against riptides. You can try, but you can also drown.

We'll discuss the relationship between chaos and order in the last section of the book, when I'll give you some tips on how to deal with this particular Fear. It's important to tackle the Fear of Chaos, because it is one of the things that introduces Stress into our lives. While we're trying to impose order on our chaos, we're not doing what we really want, or need, to do. And then resentment sets in, creating a whole new set of problems.

FEAR OF MISSING OUT: THE CAULDRON OF STRESS

"Things will go as they will; and there is no need to hurry to meet them."
—Treebeard, J.R.R. Tolkien, *The Lord of the Rings*

Directly related to the Fear of Chaos is the Fear of Missing Out.

It is one of my personal Fears. I've always had a sense that what I was doing in the moment wasn't really what I *should* be doing, that it wasn't as important as what I really *needed* or *wanted* to be doing, somewhere else.

I can't always articulate what that something else is. Sometimes I can, but more often than not, it's just a feeling, like a magnet pulling my mind into the future, to an undisclosed location, time, or activity. Many times, it prevents me from committing to a particular project or goal, because I'm afraid that if I do, I'll miss out on another opportunity.

It's pretty messed up, actually. It is at the heart of my brain-spin, my Waring Blender of Dog Shit-n-Crackers, as I like to call it. Thoughts of all the things I *should* be doing begin to swirl around in my head, waking me up in the middle of the night and interrupting my concentration during the day

When I feel that what I'm doing isn't the most important thing in that moment, I rush through it, with a feeling of angst and a pressure to finish quickly. Time seems to speed up, and I never feel I have enough of it to get done all the things I'm supposed to get done. I think it might be the cause of much of the Western World's stress. So many of us suffer from this underlying feeling that what we're doing isn't important enough to give it our full attention. Instead, our brains are spinning off into the future to work on more important tasks, or to escape work altogether.

The Illusion of Future Green Pastures

What is the root of the Fear of Missing Out? Why do we feel like there's something better, more important to do than what we're doing right now? What is pulling us away?

I think it might be linked to a belief that the future is going to be better. Most of us tend to live in the future, if we're not stuck in the past. I've found that the two work in tandem to draw my attention away from the present. There are butt-loads of Fears in the past that I project into my future, while at the same time hoping that the future will be better.

I think that my Fear of Missing Out has more to do with the Fear of Inadequacy—something we'll discuss in depth later—and the Fear of Chaos. If I don't feel that I'm good enough already, and I'm constantly worried about all the things on my To Do List, then my mind is continually drawn away to the future, where I hope that I'll be better. And maybe I can get all of those things on the list, checked off, too!

The Fear of Missing Out is like a vampire. It sucks the very life out of our existence. We become zombie-like, stumbling through life in an aimless way, staring into the future. We become disconnected from those around us because our minds aren't *here*. Instead they are drawn away to the imaginary land of *I'm good enough there*, or *Order rules there over Chaos*. We live as if we're gazing at mirages off in the desert: places that don't exist. It's a sad way to be, and I *know*! I've been there, and there are still days that I find myself zoning out, staring into space instead of engaging in the present.

There *is* nothing better out there. If we aren't present in the present, in the now, then there will *be no future*.

That's what I said.

A Zen master once said, "The future is only of any use to those who can truly live in the present." If you can't engage in the present, when you *get* to the future, you'll still be in the future! You'll never get there!

There is no future. Never was, never will be.

There is only the present. The past doesn't exist, either. It's an illusion, too.

The process of making changes in our lives can be unsettling. It brings chaos and a feeling that we're missing out. These things can grind us to a halt if we can't figure out how to deal with them. But even if we are okay with chaos, and embrace the *idea* of change, we can still be blocked if we don't know what our first step should be. If you don't know what to do *first*, how will you gain any momentum toward your goal?

FEAR OF STARTING: CATS, TREES, & PROCRASTINATION

One of the problems with change, and the process we must go through in order to affect change, is that we often don't know where to start. It's as if we are a cat stuck in a tree, uncertain of how to either get to the bird in the nest, or get back down in time for our afternoon nap.

Most of the time, when you feel stuck and afraid of starting a new change, creating a new habit, losing weight, taking a new job or looking for one, it's not because you're necessarily afraid of the outcome—though that might be part of it. Often it's because you just don't know what the first step in the process might be.

This leads to the rampant disease of *procrastination*, something most of us suffer from at some time or other. Procrastination can be caused by different Fears, but it's a symptom, not a cause. Most of the time, it's caused by not knowing what to do *first*.

Procrastination and the Fear of Starting

"What should I do first?"

If we don't know what to do first, many of us freeze, hesitate, or just give up entirely. The size of the new change and the vision of the end game is too big for us to wrap our minds around. Instead of acting, we put it off or abandon it. There is a real sense of inertia in these moments; an object at rest, tends to remain at rest. *Pass the bon bons and the Ben & Jerry's.*

Obviously, procrastination is not the road to success. The road to success is built on action. We have to pick the road, and then we have to actually *walk* down that road.

However, if you're focused too much on the outcome you'll become overwhelmed, and your mind clouded by the process you have to go through in order to achieve that end. What you need to figure out is the very first, easiest step toward achieving your goal, and take that step. We'll come back to the solution in the last chapter of the book.

If we are unable to deal with our Fears of Process, there is but one true outcome: failure to achieve our goals. And our Fear of Failure is one of the main fruits of the Fear of Outcome, the final branch of the Tree of Fear. It's a rotten limb to be sure, and we all have to walk out upon it. Will it break? Or will it hold? Keep reading, my friend.

Out on a Rotten Limb: the Fear of the Pain of Outcome
What happens if you go through all of the trouble of attempting some new thing and you fail anyway?

What happens if we take all the steps toward success, but it doesn't turn out the way we planned? What if, after working our asses off for years toward a goal, we fall flat on our faces, and don't reach it? This is a big Fear. It is the rotten, dangerous limb on the Tree of Fear that we've all been on at some point in our lives, and we dread that cracking sound. For many, the mere possibility of a negative outcome prevents them from attempting to follow their dreams. It's a weak and deadly limb but we're going out on it, anyway.

FEAR OF FAILURE

"Don't fear failure. — Not failure, but low aim, is the crime. In great attempts it is glorious even to fail." —Bruce Lee, martial arts master, and baddest of all bad asses

Of all our Fears of Outcome, the Fear of Failure is one of the most common of all. We hate to fail.

Why?

Because along with failure comes criticism, something else we hate. At the root of criticism is the Fear of Death, or annihilation.

In the Stone Ages, our ancestors were faced with death around almost every corner. Failure to kill that woolly mammoth might mean starvation for the tribe, or it might trample you into fucking dust! Failure to find suitable shelter might mean you die from exposure. Failure to find potable water or to accurately read the weather could also be deadly.

Food, shelter, and water are still essential for survival. But for most of us, they are not really a challenge anymore. We *think* they are. We *talk* as if they were still very much in question, and there is some evidence around us that we might lose them. After all, there are homeless people everywhere, even in the United States, the richest country in the world. There are also hungry people everywhere, and clean water is hard to come by in many places around the world. But for the most of us, these things are not a major challenge any longer.

Failure in the Modern World

For most of us, failure at something does not mean death. It might mean inconvenience, a major shift in occupation or the level of our creature comforts, but rarely does failure equate to death.

This Fear of Failure has become a real problem in the modern world. We have blown it out of proportion. Failure has become a dirty word and we have internalized it. If we fail at doing something, we tend to think of ourselves as being a fail*ure*: we objectify it. It moves from the verb, fail*ing*, to the noun, fail*ure*, and we identify ourselves with the noun instead of realizing that it's just a verb.

We failed at something. So what? Let's try something else! But instead, we say, *"I am a Failure,"* which is self-defeating bullshit.

Only One Way to Fail

Failing (a verb) can never make you a failure (a noun). It's impossible. That being said, you can certainly take on the appearance, of a failure. But that can only happen if you quit and *accept* failure. Einstein once said that the only way to fail was to quit trying. That doesn't mean that we can't fail. It just means that it shouldn't stop us from trying something new. Not every attempt at success will work. In fact, the vast majority of attempts *do* fail.

Most people, when faced with a daunting challenge — losing weight, exercising more, taking on a new challenge at work or a new job entirely, or leaving the so-called security of the 9 to 5 job to go into business for themselves — are stopped dead in their tracks by the Fear of Failure. In fact, this is the one that we fixate on the most, and the one we should be *least* afraid of.

Why? Because it's going to happen, and often!

Failure is unavoidable. Everyone fails, a lot. Thomas Edison, the greatest inventor of the 20th century, failed constantly. He attempted 10,000 versions of the light bulb before finding one that really worked: TEN THOUSAND. So, if you fail a couple of times, or even 9,999 times, you're ahead of Edison, and that's a pretty good place to be, if you ask me. Failure is inevitable. And it's the best teacher you're ever gonna have. In fact, it's essential to our success.

Failure is the Key to Success

If we refuse to quit, then failure isn't really failure; it's an opportunity to learn something new and move on. If Edison had been gripped by the Fear of Failure, we'd still be stubbing our toes on the way to the bathroom in the middle of the night. Before Edison, we staved off the night with torches, campfires, and oil lamps which were far more dangerous and unpredictable. Now we flip a switch, and BAM! There's light! All because he was undaunted by thousands of unsuccessful attempts.

Failure is necessary for growth. You never truly learn anything without failing. Never. Even Mozart had to learn to play a piano at some point and, as amazingly talented as he was, he most certainly was not *born* with the Magic Flute shooting out of his tiny fingertips onto the ivories. Trust me, he had to fail a lot before that happened. The same goes for Beethoven. The 9th Symphony — arguably the greatest musical work in human history — didn't happen when he was a young man; it was his *last* symphony, written after decades of work at his craft.

Failure Is Transient: Do it Quickly

Failure is almost never permanent, unless you're attempting to fly off of the top of a very tall building without a parachute; then it's pretty fuckin' permanent. Otherwise, it's just fail*ing*. The problem is when failing turns into, "I'm a fail*ure*!" Once we internalize failure, it becomes an essential part of ourselves and our story.

We are *not* failures; that's just crap. We are no such thing. If we were, we would not be able to read this book and we'd be dead. If you're not dead, you aren't a failure. Because the only way to be a failure is to *quit* trying *BEFORE* you die! If you're still busting ass when they throw the dirt on you, you rank as a success because you never, ever, ever gave in.

The way to overcome the Fear of Failure, is to ignore it altogether! We need to *embrace* failing, because it is good, helpful, and the only way to grow and learn! If we see our small, momentary failings as opportunities to stretch ourselves into something more, something bigger, then the Fear of Failure disappears.

There's a phrase in modern business that is becoming increasingly popular, "Fail fast."

What does that mean? It acknowledges that failing is just part of the process of learning, of growing, of figuring out very cool things. To fail fast, means that you learn those things that don't work, quickly, and get on to those things that do work. The faster you fail, the faster you gain clarity and can find what *does* work.

This does not mean that you can never stop and redirect your efforts. Failing is good because it helps us to change in a positive direction. Sometimes that might be a completely different direction altogether, on a different project. If you decided—after repeated failings—that a goal is unattainable in the way you were pursuing it, or that it is no longer important to you, you can always stop and change directions. That isn't quitting. In other words, we don't have to continue to chase a goal simply because we once stated it was our primary desire. Quitting is when you still want to achieve the goal, but give up because you don't think you *can* achieve it, or because it's too difficult.

But what if Failure isn't the thing holding you back? What if you're actually afraid of what might happen if you *don't* fail?

FEAR OF SUCCESS: WHAT IF THE LIMB DOESN'T BREAK?

Some people, myself included, have an even more damaging Fear than the Fear of Failure; we are afraid of what might happen if we succeed!

How fucked up is that?

Why would anyone be afraid of success?

Mostly, I think, because they haven't thought about what life would be like once they achieve it, and so they have a Fear of the Unknown, probably the most basic Fear that all living beings have. This is Lizard Brain territory, for sure.

We aren't accustomed to being successful so we find ways *not* to be. We avoid that forest altogether. We subconsciously sabotage our goals before we even start, because we have no idea what life is going to be like if we achieve them. That's pretty messed up, for sure, but true nonetheless.

That's not to say that those of us who fear success, have *never* had any success. I've achieved many things in life: academic degrees, recorded an album, published a book, written over a hundred articles, and on and on. But I've never achieved financial success, for four reasons:

1. I have a toxic relationship with money.
2. I have a Fear of Success.
3. I have a mild Fear of Failure.
4. One other Fear that we'll talk about soon.

Who Will I Be?

Another Fear driving the Fear of Success is the possible

Loss of Identity that we talked about earlier. You can see that the Fruits of the Tree of Fear can be very complex, indeed. The branches and limbs of that toxic Tree can become tangled with one another. The Fear of Success certainly belongs on the branch of Outcome, but there's also an element of Loss within that fruit.

If we actually achieve our dreams, our success, will I still be the same person? Will I become a complete douchebag like that billionaire on TV? Will money corrupt me? Will my friends and family still love me? Will I have to redefine what it means to be me? This can be unsettling.

I've actually worried if I were ever financially successful, that I would have to deal with the problem of paying my taxes! Yeah, how fuckin' ridiculous is *that*? Like I wouldn't finally be able to pay someone *else* to deal with that crap? Duh. But this is the kind of thing that can run through our brains when we're chasing a dream that we're not sure we can reach. It's also how we subconsciously set up blocks and excuses for not chasing them to begin with.

CLIMBING BACK DOWN

We could spend a lifetime picking off the nasty fruits of the Tree of Fear. But what good would that do us? Not much. We'd waste a lot of precious time and never get to the Fears that feed those fruits: the rest of the Tree. Because if you want to take down a tree, the fastest way is to start at the bottom.

So let's climb down out of this canopy and take a look at the Trunk of this twisted Tree.

TETHERED TO THE TRUNK: THE CHAINS OF OUR PAST

The problem with all of those fruity Fears at the top of our Tree isn't that there are so many of them; it's that they're all full of the same toxic sap, like the Manchineel Tree. That shit burns, stings, and can kill you if you get a good bite of it.

But that sap doesn't originate in the Fruit itself. It comes from the roots, up through the Trunk, and the further down the Tree you go, the stronger the sap. You'll also notice, as we go down the Tree, that the categories disappear; they converge near the Forest floor. That's another reason why we're going backwards. We're moving from infinitely complicated to very simple.

The Trunk is the most visible part of the Tree of Fear; it's all of those past Fears and known Fears that we constantly run into. We *know* they're there, lurking in the dark. They are Fears based on past negative experiences and they are powerful.

A Trunk with Teeth

In the Trunk, all categories of Fear exist. The Fears we *know* can be based on anything negative we've experienced in our lives. You know what those are. You don't have to think too hard to bring them back up.

In this part of the Tree lurk all the painful things that have been done to us or said about us that we actually remember in our conscious, waking mind. All forms of abuse, accidental injuries, loss of loved ones, rejections, failures, criticisms, loss of status and identity, and anything else you can think of reside in the Trunk.

The categories are the same as the ones at the top of the Tree —the future *projected* Fears—because in the past (before it *was* the past) we projected those Fears into the future which then became the past that we now remember, so we can project them all over again. How confusing is *that*? Hell, I had to take a nap after writing that sentence!

For instance, let's say that you have a really shitty boss, who, in the past, has always berated you every time you made a mistake or arrived two minutes late. She called you names and threatened to fire you or write you up every time you made the slightest error. Now, in the present, the instant you make a mistake her voice begins to ring in your ears and you experience the same physical and mental reactions you did when you saw a snake crawling across the trail in front of you in the woods.

After doing this for days, or weeks, you begin to worry that you'll make a mistake in the future—tomorrow, next week, next year—and now your Fear is out of control. Your boss is a known threat and quite possibly a real one. She is not imaginary. She could actually fire you and cause you other types of pain and fear. But you have managed to project a known Fear way out into the future, long before she *actually* threatens you. This is a very damaging type of Fear.

The Origin of the Past

The Fear of the Known is quite possibly the second major Fear that our distant ancestors developed. Way back in the mists of time, once Grandpa and Grandma had evolved from lizards to apes, they developed the part of the brain that stores memories: the Temporal Lobe (time lobe) in the middle part of our skull, just above our Lizard Brain. Let's just call it our Monkey Brain.

If, you were one of our ape ancestors, roaming the jungles of Africa some three million years ago, and you ran into lions, tigers, or bears (yeah, I know, they don't inhabit the same Eco-systems, but stay with me, I'm having fun with my Wizard of Oz analogy) then you would have experienced the Fear of the *Un*known, if it was your *first* encounter with such creatures.

If, however, you were actually attacked by them, or chased, or threatened in any way, the next time you came across the three animals from the Wizard of Oz, you would experience a new kind of Fear, one of the *Known* variety. They are no longer unknown; they are real and experienced, like your berating boss. You have catalogued them into the *dangerous* category of your ape brain and in the future, you back up to avoid them or immediately pick up a log and prepare to defend yourself if you're cornered and can't escape.

These memories of past negative experiences can serve some limited purpose if they actually keep us from returning to the same dangerous situations.

But the past only serves us if we employ it in the present to avoid possible injury—or perceived injury—in the future. But more often than not, the past holds us back because we project those painful memories into the future even when there's *no cause to do so.* Just because something happened to us once doesn't mean it will again. This constant projection of our past Fears into the future is the *poisonous sap* of the Tree, rising into the branches and fruit where it cripples us in the present because we're focused on the future.

In the final section of the book, we'll look at some techniques for chopping up the trunk of this Tree and ridding ourselves of the chain that's wrapped around it.

ROOTS IN THE DARK: TRIPPING ON THE UNKNOWN

Most of us can remember some of the painful events in our lives that left us with a sense of Fear: the death of a loved one, rejection from a lover, or a failure to achieve a goal. Those experiences can register in our brains as semi-conscious Fears that come back to block us in the present or to be projected into our future where they sabotage our chances at success.

But the trunk of the Tree is not the source of the most insidious Fears. That resides under the surface, below the dirt, in the roots and in the seed of the Tree Itself. Here we find the Fears of the *Un*known: negative experiences that happened to us long ago, often times when we were very young, and which we no longer consciously remember. They are *sub*conscious Fears. Also buried in the dirt are our basic instinctual Fears, our Lizard Brain. Let's get our shovels out and see what lies beneath the surface. Prepare to get dirty, my friends!

Fear of the Unknown

This is one that Brendon Burchard and Napoleon Hill left out. I'm not sure why or how they missed it, but it is, to me, a very important Fear.

If we encounter a stranger in a dark alley, or some new beast in the forest, we don't know whether they are actually a threat to us or not. This is when our Lizard Brain kicks in to protect us, just as it did for me when I was strolling down Queen Street so many years ago, hearing footsteps behind me. And it *did* protect me that day, for certain.

The Fear of the Unknown is probably the first fear that our most ancient ancestors—long before we were primates—must have experienced, and one that we still experience, almost daily. What we don't know can be terrifying, or at the least, unsettling. Is this new thing in front of me a threat to my life, health, or safety?

The Fear of the Unknown began as something experienced only in the present. It isn't concerned with memory or with a projection into the future; the Unknown is only concerned with clear and present dangers.

If you encounter a wild animal in the woods, a snake, for instance. What is your mental and physical reaction? Does your heart race? Your mind? Does the hair on your arms stand up? All these are Lizard Brain reactions to the Fear of the Unknown, which doesn't just manifest itself in the woods when faced with a serpent. It appears in many other forms, in our every day lives.

Fear of the Other

It's most destructive form is in a Fear of the Other. When I say 'other' I mean other humans that we don't understand: other races, cultures, languages, religions, and political views. It is this very Fear that enables every single war in the history of mankind, and many other smaller conflicts.

The Fear of the Unknown can also be a Fear of other *species* or of Nature in general. This Fear of the natural world led our species to declare war upon it with the goal of submitting it to our will, to impose our own ideas of order upon it. This was absurd, and still is. This comes from a Fear of Chaos, too. We want to smooth everything out, make it safe, predictable. But that is impossible. In the process of trying to create order in the natural world, we have destroyed much of it. If we persist, we will destroy ourselves as well as millions of other living species.

Fear of the Unknown is a deep root of the Tree of Fear but it isn't the *seed* from which the Tree is grown. There is one Fear to rule them all: the genesis of all human Fears. And that's where we're going now.

Buried in Plain Sight: the Semi-Secret Seed of the Tree of Fear

"Expose yourself to your deepest fear; after that, fear has no power, and the fear of freedom shrinks and vanishes. You are free." — Jim Morrison, rock n roll god, and dropper of massive amounts of LSD

[This is the most important chapter in the entire book. DO NOT SKIP IT! If you read nothing else, read this.]

What is the Seed of all Fear?

Where does it originate?

When I began the process of writing this book, I drew out an enormous mind-map.

If you're unfamiliar with what that is, let me explain.

A mind-map is a technique that creative people — writers, designers, programmers — use to make sense of complex ideas. It begins with brainstorming about the problem. In my case, the problem was Fear. Since it was such an enormous topic, I needed a huge canvas on which to write. I didn't have a large chalkboard or whiteboard in my house, so I rummaged around in my garage until I stumbled across one of those yard-waste bags that you put leaves and grass-clippings in.

Then I took it apart at the seams so that I could lay it out flat on my kitchen table. It covered the entire table. I then grabbed a couple Sharpies and went to work.

The way you mind-map is to just start putting topics or ideas on the page: all over it; it doesn't really matter where, unless you have a sense that a particular idea is somehow important, then you might center it, or put it at the top somewhere. Whatever you do, you don't overthink it at this point. The goal is just to get the ideas on the page and out of your head.

Then you draw lines between ideas that connect and overlap.

After a while, you start to see that some ideas have more connections than others; many lines seem to converge upon them. Those main points of convergence become chapter or section headings in the book. In my case, they were the main categories of Fear that we've been discussing.

My mind-map was enormous, and most of the lines seemed to coalesce around Loss, Process, Outcome, Unknown, Known. But I missed something in there. There was one Fear that had a lot of connections but that I overlooked on the map. When it occurred to me at first, I didn't think it was a major Fear, so I wrote it rather small and linked it under the Pain of Outcome. But I was wrong, partly. Placing it *under* Outcome was correct, but not for the reason I originally thought. By putting it in that category I had actually put it in the position of a *fruit*, not in the *roots* where it belonged.

I finally realized my mistake while watching a video by therapist, Marisa Peer, thanks to the suggestion of my coach, Bobby Kountz. Marisa was talking about an underlying negative belief we all have that drives much of our negative behavior and undermines our attempts at success and happiness.

What is this belief?

It is simply that *we are not enough*.

When I heard her say that something exploded in my head. I went running to the closet, yanked out my mind-map, spread it out on the table in the kitchen, scanned it for a few seconds, until I found it. There, in the middle of the map, in smaller scribble than the rest of the words on the page, was the word, **Inadequacy**.

I am not enough.

FEAR OF INADEQUACY: BLACK SEED OF THE TREE OF FEAR ITSELF

"Choosy mothers choose Jiff!" —popular television ad from the '70s

This, my friend, is the Seed of all Fear. It is the genesis of our Fears. It underpins all of them: the Fear of Inadequacy.

Let's think about it for a minute. What are we really afraid of when we fear Failure at work? The Process of losing weight? The Loss of a loved one? Death itself? Is it not, deep down, that we are not good enough, smart enough, knowledgeable enough, to deal with the troubles, disasters, and challenges that life throws at us? I think so.

Think of something you fear. Now dig down deep into that Fear. What do you find? What about it do you *really* fear? Isn't it that you feel inadequate to deal with the Loss, Process, or Outcome of that experience?

I think so. When I put my own Fears through this little exercise, I always come up with the same base Fear: *I am not enough to handle this, or to go through this.*

Don't believe me? Let's look at those categories again and see if my theory holds up.

Since we began with the fruits of the Tree, let's reverse it and move back up from the seed, through the roots and the trunk, to the branches.

Fear of the Unknown

What do we really Fear when we're faced with the stranger in the dark alley? With the lions, tigers, and bears? With Mr. No-Shoulders in the grass? Why should we Fear something we know nothing about? Most of the time, they turn out to be innocuous, perfectly tame and ordinary situations.

The stranger in the dark alley might be an old granny with a large shadow bringing you a basket of chocolate chip cookies. The lions, tigers, and bears might just be cowardly. Mr. No-Shoulders *might* be a very large garter snake. So, why do we fear them so much?

I think we simply question our own ability to *deal* with the unknown threat or the possible threat. We don't know, or we're convinced, that we simply aren't *good enough, smart enough, fast enough, strong enough, or bad-ass enough* to cope with the situation if it, in fact, turns dangerous.

If your name is Bruce Lee or Chuck Norris, you probably have very little Fear in a dark alley, right? If you were the late, great Crocodile Hunter, Steve Irwin, Mr. No-Shoulders would be your best friend! But most of us aren't Chuck, Bruce, or Irwin. So we feel inadequate to deal with the situation, hence the Fear. Of course, we might *not* be adequate to deal with that stranger, if it turns out *not* to be an old granny and pulls a knife on us. But how often does that happen? Not very often. What we are really feeling is our inadequacy, or our perceived inadequacy, to kick that stranger's ass if they turn violent.

Fear of the Known

This one requires less explanation. If we *know* something or someone is a threat to us, or if we failed to accomplish some goal, we already have a pretty good idea of our ability to deal with the threat or situation; we've already tested our ability.

How did we do the first time? If we failed to deal with it in the past, then our Fear of Inadequacy ramps up the next time the situation presents itself. We may fear the thing, person, or situation *itself*. The Fear of Inadequacy doesn't erase the other categories entirely, it underpins them. What we're really afraid of is that we are *still* inadequate to deal with this particular threat. We feel like a failure because we've failed in the past, *ergo*, we'll fail in the future. We *aren't good enough* to deal.

Pain of Loss

Why do we Fear it? What's at the root?

Why do we attach so much emotion to things and to other people? Why do we invest so much in them? I'm not arguing that we shouldn't love other people or be attached to them. But there's attachment that's healthy — we feel that we are enough, we contribute to their happiness and well-being, and they do the same for us. Then there's unhealthy attachment, where we don't feel enough and if they leave us we'll jump off a bridge.

The same goes for *things*. We attach ourselves and our identity to the stuff we own or want to own. I *love* this car, this house, this pair of edible underwear. We *identify* with *stuff*. Why do we do that? Why do we put so much of our own identity into other people and inanimate junk?

Because deep down, we *don't feel that we are enough*, all by ourselves.

We feel inadequate. *We aren't enough. We aren't good enough, smart enough, pretty enough, skinny enough.* We think we are lacking in all the qualities that are necessary for our own survival, and the survival of those we love. If they leave us via death, or the backdoor, or a final *text* that we get in the middle of the night, we have lost part of *who we are.* And that scares the shit out of us. How can we survive without them?

This is also true of the Fear of Rejection that Dr. Noah St. John argued was the base Fear. If we return to his example of the ancient Tribe, and put ourselves in the shoes of the tribal member in danger of being ostracized from her social group, what is her main Fear?

One might argue, that what she's really afraid of, is being rejected by the tribe, and then dying in the jungle, eviscerated and eaten by lions, tigers, and bears. But I don't think it's really *death* that she Fears. It's that she isn't capable of surviving on her own in the jungle. She simply doesn't feel that she's *good enough, strong enough, capable enough, resourceful enough,* to survive on her own. It is her Fear of Inadequacy that is at the root of her Fear of Rejection, and even her Fear of Death.

If you're Bear Grylls, you don't worry or fear a life in the jungle, forest, or tundra. You probably *love* lions, tigers, and bears. So being ostracized from your tribe, while emotionally charged and sucky, won't occasion a major Fear of Death, because you know how to survive on your own in the wild. But for most of us, rejection and a life of solitude in the forest is frightening.

Why do we Fear death anyway? Because we don't know what lies on the other side, I think. It's a Fear of the Unknown. Why do we Fear the Unknown? Because we don't feel *capable enough* to deal with something we don't know, including death itself.

Pain of Process

As already mentioned, we Fear the Pain of Process: all the crap we have to go through in order to do something new or something potentially beneficial to us. Why do we fear making changes and the process involved? Why is it a hassle? I mean, it's just *doing stuff,* right? We do stuff all the time! Why is *new* stuff so difficult?

Part of it is that it's new; it's the Unknown, which is its own Fear altogether. We don't know how it's gonna work or what the first step might be. But maybe we Fear the Process because we don't feel we're up to the challenge. In other words, we don't feel adequate for the task. We feel *in*adequate. *We aren't good enough, strong enough, willful enough, smart enough* to get through the process.

Pain of Outcome

At this point, I'm grinding up a dead stump, but I'm gonna just keep grinding it into sawdust, because this is the most important part of the entire book.

The Fear of Failure—the main Outcome we all Fear—is firmly rooted in the Fear of Inadequacy. That has become clear to me during the process of writing this book. We Fear Failure, mainly because we are sure *we aren't good enough* to succeed. We lack evidence to support the idea that we can do something extraordinary, so we take the absence of *evidence* to argue there's an absence of *ability*. But the absence of evidence is not evidence of absence.

I'm getting a bit deep there, I think. Let's see if I can write myself out of the hole.

Instead of visualizing our success, even though we have no hard evidence to support it, we instead visualize the myriad ways in which we might fail. And we are never disappointed. It's comforting to be right—remember (Fear of Being Wrong). So comforting, that we will subconsciously sabotage our own success to prove that our negative view of the world, and of our place in it, is the correct view.

How fucked up is *that*? Pretty fucked up.

But it's true. We do it. I've done it. You've done it. Everyone has done it and we continue to do it.

Inadequacy and Attraction

"But if we attract what we send out, how come that asshole over there has billions of dollars? Shouldn't he be broke like me?" you ask.

Sure, but money is just one way to measure success. What about their personal life? Their spiritual life? Their health? Their happiness? Trust me; everyone screws up at least *one* of those, if not all of them. We're all in the same boat: the U.S.S. Scared Shitless.

And it's not just failure we fear. We fear success, too! Why? Because we don't think we're *good enough, smart enough, or knowledgeable enough* to handle it! So we sabotage any success that might come our way! Remember my Fear of Success and the thoughts that ran through my head? *"If I make a lot of money doing this, how will I keep track of it? What about all the taxes I'll have to pay? Will I become a dick-head like that billionaire I saw on TV?"* I have yet to test my ability to deal with those problems. I'll get back to you on it, in another book.

This is how insidious the Fear of Inadequacy can be. It runs on autopilot, under the surface, like an evil Captain Nemo, slipping and sliding around under the waves, twenty thousand leagues under the sea of our conscious thought. We are so convinced that we're not good enough, smart enough, knowledgable enough, or pretty enough, that we don't even think it out loud much of the time. It's just kicking our ass in stealth mode.

No One is Immune: Inadequate Forest Guide?

Even I suffer from the Fear of Inadequacy.

In fact, I almost didn't write this book because I felt inadequate to do so. After all, I'm not a psychiatrist or psychologist. I'm not a sociologist or trained philosopher. I haven't spent years and decades studying people and their Fears, not professionally anyway. What could I *possibly* contribute to such an enormous topic? Even the professionals I've mentioned haven't attempted to do what I'm doing here in this book. Why not?

I would suggest that they haven't done it for one of two reasons. One, they haven't actually thought of Fear in quite this way. Two, they stopped short due to their own Fears of Inadequacy, or of Criticism (a very high likelihood, given the contentious nature of academia), or of Loss, especially of loss of status or their position in the professional community.

All during the process of writing this book, and especially near the end, I was plagued by the Fear that it just *wasn't good enough*. Despite what skills and knowledge I might have, the book simply wan't good enough. I would put it out into the world, but maybe it wouldn't resonate with anyone.

What if no one likes it?

What if it helps no one?

What if I never write a book that succeeds?

Why should anyone follow me through this Forest, if I can't even find the path?

What good am I as a guide, if I'm paralyzed listening to wolves?

All these Fears came flooding into my mind one night, waking me up at 2 a.m. with the Whirlpool of Piss I mentioned earlier in the chapter about the Wolves of Debt. The Fears stopped me in my tracks, right in the middle of the darkest part of the Forest, where wolves howl, bears prowl, and evil witches boil and bubble, toil and trouble. It is *not* a place anyone wants to be. But I managed to keep moving, because the book is in your hands.

Devourer of Dreams

This Fear of Inadequacy kills dreams, it kills success, it kills relationships, and it kills people. It swallows them whole, like the Big Bad Wolf did to Grandma and Little Red Riding Hood.

Think about the last time you thought about looking for a new job. What were your concerns? Did you think, "I'd really like to make more money and move into that new field of work but I don't think I'm qualified for that position or that level of work"? *Don't think I'm qualified* translates into *I'm not good enough, smart enough, knowledgeable enough*.

Now, it might be true that you don't yet possess the knowledge to do a particular job that you aspire to. But that was true of the person who is *now* doing the job. How did they gain the knowledge? In high-school? In college? Not likely and not usually. Most people learn to do their job *ON THE JOB!* Most jobs require you to know stuff that just isn't taught anywhere else. You simply have to *do it* to *learn it*. It has absolutely nothing to do with knowing it beforehand.

The *not smart enough* or *not good enough* parts of our thought process are simply bullshit. They are in our own head. If we can conceive of doing it we are capable of doing it. There are people with severe mental and physical, so-called *handicaps* out there, doing amazing things with their minds and bodies. So there *is no* 'not good enough', or 'not smart enough.' It's bullshit. It's our own Fear of Inadequacy.

Who Planted This Damned Seed?

Who was the Johnny Appleseed of Inadequacy?

Where did we get this destructive Fear?

Short answer? We learned it.

Mostly, our parents taught us to feel less than enough.

Why? Because their parents taught it to them. But they weren't our *only* instructors in Inadequacy 101. Our entire society, even civilization itself, is built upon the very idea that we are not enough. *We are small, insignificant cogs in a very large machine and there's nothing we can do about it.* That has been the prevailing myth in the Western World for a long time unless you count the even older myth: we're all just pawns of a celestial monarch. Either way, we're not good enough or all that significant. The message is basically the same. And it isn't just cold-hard science or benevolent authoritarian religion that tells us this. Our new religion, Capitalism, is based firmly on the belief that we're all inadequate, unless we bow to Wall Street or at least go shopping.

All advertising is built upon the Fear of Inadequacy. Look around you. Find a handful of ads from TV, radio, or print, and look for the underlying message.

What is it?

It's all Freudian, Fear-based persuasion based on our Fear of Inadequacy:

You are not good enough, UNLESS, *you purchase this new dress, this new-and-improved cereal, this new car, this big-as-fuck-house-that-you-can't-actually-afford. You are a lousy, worthless mother, if you don't feed your kids this sugar-coated cereal, or take them to McDonald's every day for a fucking Happy Meal. Remember! Choosy Mothers choose Jiff! Why? Because if you don't, you suck at motherhood and your children are going to die of embarrassment when their friends find out their eating that knock-off brand!*

That is the message, loud and clear. We aren't good enough unless we buy a bunch of crap that we don't need and, most of the time is toxic to our very survival. And we've bought the lie, hook, line, and sinker.

Why?

Because we already believed it. We've been conditioned since birth to believe in our own limitations and inadequacies. That's why it's so easy to sell us stuff we don't need, because we really, truly *believe* that we *do need it*. We aren't good enough without it.

I call Bullshit.

We *are good enough*.

YES WE ARE!!

The Fear of Inadequacy is the Gordian Knot, the Black Seed of Fears. If we can unravel IT, if we can dig it up and expose it to the sun, we might just unravel the rest. Get rid of the Seed and the rest of the Tree will come crashing down to the Forest floor.

It's time to stop cataloging Fears and start eradicating them! You ready for some Lumberjacking? Get your flannel shirt, pull on your dungarees and some heavy boots and sharpen your axe. We're gonna cut a path to the Tree and bring that bastard down!

GOODIE BASKET FOUR: ANATOMY OF FEAR

- **There are Six major categories of Fear:**
    - Pain of Loss
    - Pain of Process
    - Pain of Outcome
    - Known Fears
    - Unknown Fears
    - Fear of Inadequacy
- **The Fear of Inadequacy** is the Seed of the Tree of Fear. From it, all Fears spring.

5

You're a Lumberjack and You're Okay

DO YOU HAVE THE POWER TO END FEAR ITSELF?

"We but mirror the world. All the tendencies present in the outer world are to be found in the world of our body. If we could change ourselves, the tendencies in the world would also change. As a man changes his own nature, so does the attitude of the world change towards him. This is the divine mystery supreme. A wonderful thing it is and the source of our happiness. We need not wait to see what others do." – Mahatma Gandhi, anti-violent leader, philosopher, and home-made toga-maker

"What can one person do to change a world filled with so much hate, violence, intolerance, and Fear?"

That's a very good question with a very simple answer: a whole shit-ton. The impact of one person can be, and often is, massive. Each of us has the capacity to affect enormous change in the world if we simply *believe* we can. The examples are too numerous to list.

We *do* have the power. We just don't *think* we do, and then we don't *act*. It's much easier to default to one of the other myths — *there are too many problems, it's human nature, Fear is good for me, Fear is too complicated* — and do nothing. But that won't solve the problems. The only reason we *can't* solve the world's problems is because we have a Fear that we are powerless to do so, and that my friend is complete and utter bullshit.

The beauty is that we don't have to End Fear Itself for everyone. In fact, we can't. We have no power to change someone else: not one bit. We must begin with what we *do* have the power to change: ourselves. In fact, that's really all we *can* change. Until we get a handle on our own Fears, how can we expect to help anyone else with theirs?

Do you possess the power to bring down the Tree of Fear Itself?

The answer to this question is *you're damned right you do*. In fact, YOU are the only person on Earth with the power to end Fear Itself. That's because in order to end Fear Itself each individual must look inward into their own Fears, to their own Tree of Fear, and do the work to bring it down.

You must kick your own ass.

I said it.

Your Fears are destroying your life, turning you into a pathetic, weak, zombie-like creature, lumbering around, brainless and directionless, waiting for the shot-gun blast, or the swing of a cricket bat to end your suffering. And if you're not quite that pathetic, then your Fears are, at a minimum, blocking you from the success you've always wanted.

Fuck that!

It's time to pull up our big-boy/big-girl pants and face those Fears head on.

In the next few chapters, we'll dive deep into some of these Fears and see how we can give them a swift kick out the door.

You ready?

TAKING DOWN THE FEAR TREE: EXPOSING SEEDS & ROOTS

"If a fear cannot be articulated, it can't be conquered." —Stephen King, author and master of Fear

The first step to overcoming Fear is to identify the ones that are holding you back from what you want to achieve.

I'm assuming—since you're reading this book—that you realize that you have some limiting Fears in your life.

That's good.

It's the first step.

You might even have some pretty good ideas about what those Fears are. But I suspect, if you're like me, there are some Fears buried in your conscious and subconscious mind that are even more damaging, especially the subconscious ones.

We began our look at the categories of Fear with what I called the *fruits* of the poisoned Tree (or Projected Fears). Then we worked our way downwards, through the *branches* (Loss, Process, Outcome), the *trunk* (Known) and into the *roots* (Unknown), and we ended up by uncovering the Seed of all Fear: the Fear of Inadequacy.

There was a method to my working in that downward direction. I was attempting to *un*explain Fear. The problem with a topic as large as Fear is that it seems entirely too complicated to ever tackle. That's because we spend most of our time staring at all the leaves and fruits on the tree. We can't see the Tree for the Forest, to use an old metaphor and turn it around. We're staring at the forest, the leaves and fruits, and there are just too many of them.

But if you want to get rid of the leaves and the fruits of your personal Manchineel Tree, then you don't start picking fruits off of it with the idea that you'll eventually get them all. That would take forever and, while your hands were burning and blistering from contact with each and every fruit and leaf, the Tree would replace them almost as fast as you could harvest them. You'd never finish and you'd be dead long before you got to the branches, let alone the trunk, roots, and seed.

Instead, let's just go for the seeds and roots to begin with: the Unknown stuff. We have to make them *known* before we can really deal with them. Once they're out in the light of day, we can destroy them in short order.

When we're done with those, we'll deal with any remaining fruits that might be lying around on the ground. They'll be easier to deal with after cutting the Tree down, and most of them will dissipate in the process of swinging the axe.

First, let's break out our shovels and start digging for roots.

What You'll Need:

- *Patience*: This is not a quick fix. It took decades to grow this Tree. It won't come down in an instant.

- *Pen and Paper*: I would suggest actually writing this stuff down, longhand, in a journal, on a legal pad, whatever works for you. Writing longhand has a magical connection to the subconscious. But if you prefer, type it, or record it via voice.

- *Time, Space, and Silence*: While you could, theoretically, do these exercises in a crowded disco club, I wouldn't recommend it. Find a space where you can think without distractions. Put the cell phone in another room, on *silent*. Turn off the computer screen and the TV. Music is okay as long as it doesn't distract you.

SHOVELING DOWN: QUESTIONING UP THE UNKNOWN

The best way to get to the roots of your Fear Tree is to start with a question.

For years I've always told my friends that the most dangerous thing in the world is a question. The human mind is built to answer them. Our subconscious mind can't ignore them for long. Once we hear a question our minds go to work on them. And they always come back with some kind of answer. The answer might not always be correct, but the answers always come. If you want to know what Fears lie hidden in your subconscious, all you have to do is ask.

One of the best questions I've come across to get to those Fear roots, is the following:

"What am I *not* doing right now, that I know I want to, need to, or should do?"

If there's something you really want to do, but aren't doing, Fear is at the root of the 'why.' It's *always* there. It might be a Fear that you already know but, more often than not, there are also a couple of hidden Fears behind those things we aren't doing. If you want to succeed in life—however you define success, in whatever area of your life—then you *must* identify, and deal with, those Fears. If you don't, you'll never be successful in that area.

How It Works
Ask yourself the following question about every major area of

your life:

"*What do I need to be doing to achieve success in* <u>(fill in the blank)</u> *area of my life, right now, that I'm not currently doing?*"

It could be something pertaining to your health, like eating better — one of my *ain't doings* — or your work/business, or your personal life.

What you're going to find is, that behind all of your *not doings*, is a Fear, or more than one. Try to identify them. Put a name on them. Then you can start to dispel them, over time, with the techniques in the following sections of the book. Sometimes the act of shining a light on them is enough.

List the following areas of your life on a legal pad, in a journal, or computer document, and use the shovel question to identify any blocking Fears that are keeping you from success in each one of the areas. Don't rush through this step. It might only take you 20 minutes, but it could take you days if you're really blocked or have a lot of Fears. It's okay if it takes awhile. It's not a race, my friend. Take your time and dig up the things that are preventing you from being the *you* you want to be.

Here are the areas to focus on:

1.   Spiritual/Religious/Purpose
2.   Health/Physical Well-being
3.   Personal Time
4.   Relationships
5.   Work/Business
6.   Financial

Work through each of them, starting with your inner, spiritual well-being and purpose. It is the cornerstone of your life. You don't have to be religious to have a spiritual connection with the people and things around you. And you don't have to think of it in a hippy dippy way. Just think of it as finding your purpose or mission in life. That's all.

Your Spiritual Life/Life Purpose

What do you know you need to do to improve your connection with your inner spirit, with God, your religion (if you have one)? Why aren't you currently doing this? What's holding you up? Have you ever considered what your purpose in life might be? If not, then it's time to start. What's keeping you from doing *that*?

Your Health

What are you not doing right now that would improve your health, your fitness? Are you exercising regularly? And I don't mean running marathons or lifting weights every day. That's not necessary, despite what our culture and most doctors will tell you. The key to a long life is really just moderate exercise, done a little every day.

How about your diet? Are you eating enough veggies? I don't. This is one I'm still working on, so this paragraph is for Steve Bivans and anyone else out there like me. Why aren't we eating our veggies? Very good question.

Personal Time

Do you take personal time? Do you take vacations away from work, your business? Each week? Every year? If not, why? Personal time, away from work and the stress of building a business or running a household, is essential. It helps us to recharge our batteries. Our minds and spirits really do work like D-cell batteries, my friend. If you don't recharge them every once in a while, they will run down and start to ooze acid all over the place, metaphorically speaking of course. And no one wants that! So, what is holding you back from taking time off? What Fear is behind it?

Your Relationships

So often, we neglect our closest relationships because we take them for granted. We don't spend time working on them to make them stronger. What do you know you could be doing, right now, to strengthen the relationship you have with your spouse or partner? What about your children, if you have any? Your parents? The rest of your family? What about your friends? Are you spending time with them? Why not? What are you afraid of? (Hint: It might be the Fear of Chaos)

Your Work, Your Business

This is the one category that we usually worry about the most. Some of us think we have an idea of what we could be doing to improve our workplace, the work we do there, or how to better build up our businesses. But often we aren't doing those things. What do you think you could be doing right now to make your work or your business run smoother, be more productive, less chaotic, and more profitable? Why aren't you doing it? What Fear is lurking behind that, and *why*?

Your Finances

This is a tough one for me. I've struggled with money my entire adult life, due largely, I'm sure, to the attitudes I picked up about money when I was a child. But I'm working on it these days. I still have a lot of work to do and some of that I've been putting off. Why? Because I have Fears about doing that work, especially the *process* of doing it. I have Fears about the whole topic of Finances.

What do *you* need to do to get your financial life in order? Take a hard look at your debts? Make a plan to deal with them? Create a budget and follow it? Find new revenue streams? Cut unnecessary expenses? Why aren't you doing it? What Fear do *you* have around the topic of money?

Take each of these categories, one at a time, and really think about what is holding you back from doing the things you want, or need to do, to improve on them. This takes some real thought. But DON'T SKIP THIS STEP! If you do, then the entire book will be a waste, because you can't end Fear, if you don't know WHAT YOU FEAR.

You must take some time to figure out what it is that you're afraid of, if you really want to make positive changes, and be successful in each of these areas of your life. Some people are very successful and less fearful in one or more aspects of their life; maybe you're one of them. That's awesome. But there must be at least one area that you really need to work on or you wouldn't be reading this book. My bet is that there are Fears lurking under the surface in all areas of your life. Take the time to dig them out. It's worth the effort.

Excavating the Seed of Fear

How did your Fear-digging exercise go?

Were you able to uncover some Unknown or Known Fears that are blocking you from succeeding in major areas of your life?

If you haven't gone through the shovel question exercise, then you better get to work on it, or the rest of this book won't help you much. Of course, you can keep reading through if you want, but make sure to go back and actually *implement* the ideas and *do* the exercises. Otherwise, you wasted your money on this book. An intellectual understanding of Fear won't bring an end to it.

Seed Diggin'

As you know, the Seed of the entire Tree of Fear is the Fear of Inadequacy. If you have even the slightest hint of it in your mind, you will find that success in one or more areas of your life will be nearly impossible.

Look back at the answers to the question you posed in the last section.

Do you see any versions of *"I am not enough"* in your answers?

It tends to show up in the following ways, but isn't limited to these:

- I'm not smart enough.
- I don't know if I'm a very good parent, spouse, friend, employee, etc…
- I'm not qualified for (a particular job, position, business).
- I don't feel comfortable asking for more money, because….
- I'm too fat.
- I'm not pretty enough.
- I'm too old, or too young to do _____.
- I don't know how to do ____.

- I don't have enough training to do _____.
- I don't feel confident enough to do _____.

If you don't see any of these, I would challenge you to dig into the Fears you *did* find, and see if you can dig deeper into them. Most of the time, the Fear of Inadequacy manifests itself as a version of one of the above statements, either as a thought in the mind or spoken out loud.

Once you spot any of these, you know that the Seed of Fear exists in your life. If you really want to succeed, you need to dig it out and kill it. But it's helpful, once you identify a Fear of Inadequacy in a particular area, to examine it a little further. This will help you to reprogram your mind in the next step of the process.

Ask yourself the following questions about your Fears of Inadequacy:

- Where did this Fear of Inadequacy originate? Dig down deep into your Past experiences to find our where it comes from.
- Who planted this seed in your mind?
  - Your parents?
  - Other relatives?
  - Teachers?
  - Friends?
  - Enemies?

Go through all of your Shovel Down Answers and pose these questions to any instances where there's a hint of *I'm not enough*. It might be that the Fear of Inadequacy only appears in one area of your life or it might exist in all of them. Either way, work through each area asking yourself, 'Where did this originate?' and 'Who planted it?' Write it all down in your journal. We're gonna use that information to go after that seed with a vengeance. Let's get started!

WHY ARE YOU ENOUGH?: KILLING THE SEED WITH QUESTIONS

From Inadequacy to Confidence

The best way to deal with the Fear of Inadequacy, the Fear that I'm Not Good Enough, is to come to the realization that you really *are* good enough.

This is a tough one that I'm currently working on myself. As confident as I might seem, there's always a part of me that thinks, *"Who the hell am I to be writing this stuff? What authority do I really have to do it?"* But thanks to my coach, Bobby Kountz, and a video he turned me onto, I'm beginning to realize that I *am* good enough.

A couple months ago, Bobby texted me a link to a video by famed, therapist, Marisa Peer, who has worked with thousands of clients in the entertainment and sports world for a couple decades or more. In her YouTube video, *The Biggest Disease Affecting Humanity: "I'm not enough."* she suggests that our Fear of Inadequacy —*we're not enough*—is the biggest stumbling block to our happiness and success. I agree. When I saw the video, it hit me like a ton of bricks. My earliest discussions on the topic of Fear, with my friend Justin Finkelstein, were on that very subject.

When I watched the video, I suddenly realized that this entire book had to be rearranged. The very *Seed* of all Fears, is our Fear of Inadequacy and that if we want to bring about the End of Fear Itself we have to start by eliminating that deadly seed.

How do we do that? The Power of Words

So how do we even *begin* to turn around our own limitations? Our Fear of Inadequacy?

We do it with the power of words.

When I tell you the solution you're gonna think I'm nuts because it's just too simple to work. But it does, in fact, work.

Ms. Peer uses a couple of techniques with her clients. I'm sure that if you were one of her private clients, you'd get to lie down on her couch where she'd employ hypnosis to reprogram your subconscious directly. Of course, for most of us that isn't an option. The other method she suggests involves the use of positive affirmations.

Marisa tells several stories in her lecture of clients who used positive affirmations—positive statements—to reprogram their subconscious away from all of those negative thoughts of Inadequacy—*I'm not good enough.* Basically, she told them to go around their house and write *I Am Enough* on every mirror—with lipstick—and to program their phones to send them messages throughout their day to tell them the same thing: *I Am Enough.*

I actually tried this. It had some noticeable effect, for sure. Many of Marisa's clients have experienced dramatic, life-changing results from this method. But for many people, positive affirmations just aren't enough to get the job done and there's a really logical reason why.

We simply don't believe them.

The Problem With Positivity

Have you ever received a complement?

Has anyone ever said, "You're really beautiful!" or "You're amazing!" or "You did such an awesome job on that!"?

Of course they have. All of us have received praise at some point in our lives, probably thousands of times. But what was your reaction?

Was it:

"Whatever..."

"Yeah, sure..."

"It wasn't that big a deal..."?

Most likely. Most of us really hate getting praise, even though we crave it like mad.

Why is that?

We hate it because we don't feel worthy of it. We have a Fear of Inadequacy so we don't believe people when they say nice things about us, especially *to* us. It makes us uncomfortable because, deep in our subconscious, we don't feel that the compliments are true. We simply don't believe them.

For most of us, the same thing applies to positive affirmations.

This is not to say that affirmations don't work at *all*. They do for some people, some of the time. But for many people, myself included, they have limited to little effect because as soon as we say to ourselves, "I am enough," our subconscious replies with heavy sarcasm, "Yeah, whatthefuck ever."

There's a gap of disbelief. Our minds simply *know* the statement is untrue, contrary to fact. It creates a cognitive dissonance, a disharmony of the brain, that tells us it's complete bullshit.

So how do we bridge this gap of disbelief? The answer is in the question.

The Power of the Right Question

Remember at the beginning of the last section when I was explaining the power of questions on the subconscious mind? Well, we're going to return to that, probably several times before we reach the end of this book because nothing is more powerful than a question except possibly the power of moving water. But water-boarding isn't all that useful to removing Fear, I'm told, so we'll stick with probing questions.

For a month or so, I've been trying Marisa Peer's method of positive affirmations, and they've had some noticeable effect. But it hasn't been dramatic, especially in the area of money. I simply can't seem to get my subconscious to accept *"I am rich,"* or *"I have buttloads of money."* My brain shoots right back, *"Oh hell no you ain't! Have you looked at your bank account lately?"* The reality brick drops on my toe and the Law of Attraction is thrown in reverse.

But just recently, I ran across a book, *Demons in the Celler* by Tim Ebl, a fellow author in my Self-Publishing School Mastermind Group. In it, Tim suggests that a better method than affirmations is to simply turn them into *questions*. For instance, instead of *"I Am Enough,"* it would be *"Why am I Enough?"* This also hit me like a ton of bricks, since it resonated with my long-held belief that there was nothing more powerful than a question.

The next day, Bobby Kountz told me to read *The Book of Affirmations©* by Dr. Noah St. John. The entire thesis of the book is exactly what Tim Ebl said in his book, and what I'm getting ready to tell you now. If you really want to reprogram your subconscious, quickly, then don't TELL it what to think, ASK it *why* you're already there.

What do I mean?

Well, Dr. St. John pioneered this technique almost 20 years

ago. And he argues that the subconscious mind cannot ignore probing questions, especially those that start with *'why'*. Why is a very powerful word. It gets to the root of meaning, of purpose. Other question words like 'how,' and 'what,' are useful for some purposes, but in Dr. St. John's opinion, 'why' is the most effective.

He suggests that if we really want to change our negative subconscious programming, the best way is to ask ourselves 'why' questions.

Here's the Exercise:

- Take out your journal, or a piece of paper.
- **Write, *Why am I Enough?***
- Read it out loud.
- Twice, daily, before bed and when you wake up, read it out loud again.
- Make a recording of it, over and over again, on your *voice memo* app on your phone, or on your computer, and listen to it for several minutes each day.

You can use many variations on the same question: *why am I so awesome?; Why do I kick ass?; Why am I so fuckin' amazing? (one of mine)*. Or, you can get Dr. St. John's book, read the whole thing and find many more suggestions in the last series of chapters. I'll give you a few more of my own questions in later sections.

Afformations© can be used to reprogram ALL of your Fears, not just Inadequacy.

The reason this technique works is because we're already doing it. As Dr. St. John points out, we do it all the time, except that we ask the wrong questions: *negative* questions.

"Why am I always broke?"

"Why am I so stupid?"

"Why do I always fail?" and on and on and on.

Our brain works very hard to answer all those negative questions and it does a very good job of it. It comes back with answers like,

"Because you're lazy, or unlucky, or it's the economy's fault, or the

government's fault" or

"Because you never do anything right, and your whole family is stupid," or

"Because you're not smart enough to succeed."

And the answers keep coming.

Wouldn't it be better to just ask ourselves some positive questions?

A Friendly Reminder

One of the difficult things about doing any self-help stuff is remembering to actually *do* it during our ridiculously busy lives. So, I'm gonna give you a tip on a very cool smart-phone app called **HiFutureSelf**.

HiFutureSelf has a free version with limited function. I would strongly suggest you get the 'pro' version, which is only like $3 or $4, and totally worth it. The app is a simple calendar-based tool to help remind you of important dates and times. You could probably set Google Calendar up to do it but HiFutureSelf is simpler to use.

Here's what you do:

Whenever you create a new positive question you want to ask your subconscious, you program it into HFS to pop up on your phone at a certain time during the day. In the pro version, you can program it to repeat: every hour, once a day, once a week, month, etc. I suggest that the first thing you program in, is some version of *"Why am I enough?"* and that you set it to come up once every hour, of every day, at least for a week or so. Then you can back it down, or ask the question in a different way.

Change It Up

You do want to change up your questions because after a while the brain gets used to a particular question and begins to ignore it. The brain ignores the usual and focuses on what is new. So come up with new ways to ask positive questions and keep them fresh.

Dr. St. John's clients have had amazing results with his method and he's been doing it for over 20 years. But don't forget Marisa Peer's method, too. Electronic reminders are great, but make sure to put the message where you'll see it in the physical world, as well.

Ask yourself, *"Why am I so amazing?"*

- Write it on your bathroom mirror!
- Write it on your living room mirror!
- Print it out and tape it on your fridge, next your kid's crayon artwork!
- Create a background for your computer screen and put it as your wallpaper! (this is a very good one)
- Get a tattoo! Maybe on your forehead so you can see it in the mirror? (One of Marisa's followers actually *did* get a tattoo, but on her hand, not forehead)

With these methods you can dig up that nasty Seed: the Fear of Inadequacy and leave it out in the sun till it dries up and blows away!

Axe to Trunk: Felling the Tree of Fear

Once you've identified the things you Fear, the Roots of your Fear of Inadequacy, and the roots of other known Fears, or previously unknown ones, you can the start to chop down this poisonous Tree with a toolbox of special axes:

THE AXE OF AFFORMATIONS©

The tool of positive Afformations© —those questions that Dr. St. John suggested —works just as well on all of your other Fears as it did on the Fear of Inadequacy. Once you've identified a particular root Fear, or fruit Fear for that matter, you can apply positive questions to it to reprogram your subconscious to think in a new, positive, non-fearful way.

For example, let's say you have a Fear of Failure, one of the Outcome Fears. You can compose some positive questions to flip the Fear around. The way to do this is to write the question in such a way which assumes what you want —the desired outcome —has already happened. So, instead of *"I always fail,"* it would be *"Why do I always succeed?"* or *"Why did I succeed at (something you aspire to achieve)?"*

Some examples:

- *Why am I so successful?*
- *Why did I achieve _____?*
- *Why am I so rich? wealthy?*
- *Why do I always have more money than I need?*
- *Why am I so resourceful?*
- *Why does everyone love me?*

- *Why did I lose 20 lbs by (fill in the blank with a future date)?*
- *Why am I so beautiful?*

The list is endless. You can come up with thousands of your own. And do it for every area of your life, from rebuilding self-confidence, to your work, business, finances, health, and your relationships.

My suggestion is to pick one of those areas, the one you need to work on the most, and start there. The best way to do it is to catch yourself in your negative self-talk mode and then flip the negative statement or question into a positive one. Keep doing this, gradually adding new Afformations© into each area of your life, mixing them up occasionally so they don't get stale. Over time, nearly everything you think and say will be positive!

If there's ONE tool in this book that will do the most to help transform your life, this is probably it. The rest of the tools are great, and will help, but I don't think any of them have the power that this one does. So pick up that axe and swing away!

THE AXE OF FORGIVENESS:

"People are often unreasonable, illogical and self centered; Forgive them anyway." — Mother Teresa

As we talked about in the Fear of the Known section, some Fears are related to negative experiences that we *know* we've had in our Past. Maybe you were abused as a child or as an adult. This can be either physical or verbal. Both are destructive as hell. They plant all kinds of negative affirmations in our minds.

Of course, not all negative experiences are abuse. Many are just things that went wrong in our lives, or bad choices we made, or goals that we failed to achieve, or people that rejected us. Negative experiences come to us in infinite ways.

Sometimes we forget that they ever happened; they become Unknown Fears, lodged in our subconscious. This is where our Fear of Inadequacy originates.

Once you dig them out with the Shoveling Down Questions, they become *known* Fears, which are much simpler to address. *Simple* does not mean *easy*, however. Dispelling Fear is difficult work, even if the concept is simple to understand. A great way to deal with Fears which we know originate from interactions with other people is to practice forgiveness.

Forgiveness is For the Forgiver

"But some people just don't deserve to be forgiven!"

It's hard to forgive some people for the hurt they've done to us. I get it. I've carried around anger and resentment towards people for years. But in the last few years, I've tried to let all that go. Why? Because it doesn't harm *them*; it only harms *me*! If you hold hatred towards someone who abused you, or wronged you in the past, no matter what the nature of that abuse was, who does it really harm? Answer: YOU!

Chances are, the person you hate doesn't even know it, or if they do, they don't think about your hatred very much. Why? Because if you hate them, most of the time you don't bother to talk to them, so they're not continually reminded of your feelings towards them. But *you are*! You live with it all the time, or at least every time you think of them. My hatred used to ruin whole days for me every time I thought of a particular couple of people. How ridiculous is that?

Forgiveness isn't really *for* the forgiven; it's for the forgiv*er*. It's for you. It's for your own sanity, happiness, and success. You'll never be wholly successful if you're carrying around hatred and resentment for something someone else did to you.

Give it up already, and feel the weight drop from your own mind and body.

Forgiving Yourself

And while you're at it, don't forget to forgive your*self*!

So many of our negative experiences are caused by our own mistakes and our own bad choices. Sometimes we just fall on our face. Shit happens. We don't always succeed in the pursuit of our goals. Sometimes we let other people down. Most of the time, we just let ourselves down. And that's a tough one to deal with.

You know what? Get over it.

Forgiveness is for the forgiver, remember? So, forgive *yourself*, too! Not because your Failure Self deserves it, but because *you* need it. I know that's confusing, but it's true. Don't leave yourself out when it comes to forgiveness or all the effects of forgiving everyone else will be greatly diminished, if not rendered completely pointless.

The following method for forgiveness comes from Tim Ebl's book, *Demons in the Cellar*, which is all about overcoming the Fear and negative emotions surrounding abuse. It works for forgiving anyone. That includes forgiving yourself for forgetting to take out the garbage last night. I offer this stripped down basic version of it, here. He goes into way more detail, if you want it. I definitely recommend his book.

Ebl's Forgiveness Formula:

1. **Bring to mind** someone who has wronged you, or something you failed to do, or something you did that hurt someone else.

2. **Write an apology letter**, from them to YOU. Make them beg for forgiveness and make it detailed. Or, write an apology letter to yourself for any failures on your part, or to someone else, if you feel you need to apologize to someone. (You don't have to send it)

3. **Read it out loud** to yourself, then take a break, maybe for a day or two or more.

4. **Write a letter** to them, forgiving them. Or write a letter *from* them, or from yourself, forgiving yourself for what you did, or failed to do. Also make it detailed.

5. **Read it out loud** to yourself.

6. **Then let it go.** From now on, the feelings are on YOU.

Do this as many times as you need, for every person that has wronged you, or for every time you've wronged someone else, or let yourself down.

If you do this, you will no longer be a victim in the situation.

You will be in control, and you can let go of all the Fear, anger, and hatred that you have built up inside, which is only killing YOU.

Storytelling: a Two Bladed Axe

"Fear, to a great extent, is born of a story we tell ourselves..." Cheryl Strayed, author

One of the most powerful tools we can use to chop up our Fears is our Story Axe. That's because everything we think about our life is simply the story we tell about it. *We* write it, every day, every minute. And there is no more powerful story on Earth, for each of us, than our own story. It determines everything we think about the world. But there are two sides to that Story Axe, so be careful how you swing it.

Blade One: Tragedy

"Battle Stations! Battle Stations!" boomed the voice of Commander Kyes over the intercom.

Fireman Second Class, Ray Felt, leaped from his bunk where he had been sleeping for only an hour or so and sprang into action. At 0210 hours, 2:10 a.m., minutes after Ray had been so abruptly awakened, an explosion rocked the ship. This was followed, five seconds later, with another. Twenty-seven minutes later a third explosion completed the job. The ship was doomed.

Ray Felt passed away the week I was writing this chapter, at the age of 93. He grew up a farm boy in rural Minnesota in the 1920s and '30s, during the Great Depression—no shortage of Fear during that period—and when WWII came, he signed up for the Navy, and was assigned to the destroyer U.S.S. Leary.

Fear, or at least fear*ing*, was just part of the job, and the threat of German U-boats in the Atlantic was palpable, and real. Hundreds of ships had already been sent to Davy Jones's Locker before Ray's ship was assigned Task Group 21.41 to escort the aircraft carrier U.S.S. Card in a hunt for a pack of wolves—dreaded U-boats—hundreds of miles of the coast of Spain and Portugal.

On December 24th, Christmas Eve 1943, they found the wolves, or the pack found them. Commander Kyes sounded battle stations but before the Leary could locate the U-boats, at 0210 hours, two torpedoes rocked the ship's engine room, instantly killing everyone in that section of the ship and leaving the Leary dead in the water: no engines, no navigation—a sitting target. And we already know what happens to those who sit still in wolf territory.

The inevitable followed; another German torpedo slammed into the side of the listing Leery, splitting her up as the captain yelled for all hands to "abandon ship!" Ray and his friends—those not killed in the blast or trapped below deck, did just that; they jumped overboard into the icy cold Atlantic. Luckily for Ray, he was wearing a lifejacket.

Ray and his mates, only 200 yards from the doomed vessel, watched as the burning, smoking Leery disappeared below the waves "in a mighty roar," along with 98 of their friends and fellow sailors, including their brave Commander Kyes. A tragic tale if ever there was one.

The Other Side of the Axe: Courage and Compassion

When a hundred men go down with a ship, it is a massive loss, no matter how you want to look at it. I would never argue otherwise. In that number were boys no older than 17 or 18, and probably a few who were 15 or 16 who lied about their age so they could avenge the sneak attack on Pearl Harbor. There were also men with families: wives, children, mothers, fathers, aunts and uncles. There is no way to calculate or measure the loss to those families. There never is.

But loss is only one side of the story. There is also heroism, courage, compassion, and friendship in this story, and every single story about war, in every period of history.

The last act of brave Commander Kyes was to give his lifejacket to one of his crew before going down with his ship, never to be seen again. One man giving his life for another: the ultimate sacrifice. There isn't much one can do in life that is more beautiful than that. One man made it home to his family that would not have. Others did, as well, thanks to the bravery and compassion of their brothers in arms.

The survivors of that wolf attack, Ray among them, floated in the frigid waters for hours upon hours before another ship from the task force could reach them to pull them out. By that time, Ray had passed out from hypothermia, According to him, he would never have survived without the two friends floating next to him who kept his head above water until he was snatched from the jaws of the Atlantic—friendship and compassion.

Thanks to those two friends, Ray made it home and survived the war. He and his wife adopted two children and lived to see several grandchildren grow up to have children of their own. Without the aid of his friends that day in the icy Atlantic, three generations of the Felt family would never have been born. I would not be sitting in a home with one of them writing this book. It is quite possible that I might never have been inspired to write it at all.

One of the things that happens in war is that thousands, sometimes millions, of men and women leave home and family behind, to kill each other. But the other thing that also happens, is that men, women, and children, perform extraordinary acts of kindness, charity, compassion, courage, and self-sacrifice all for the sake of their shared humanity, even, many times, for those whom they are fighting against.

While war—or suffering of any kind—isn't beautiful in and of itself, there is always beauty, usually in the form of Courage and Compassion, following in its wake. You just have to look for that story. It's always there.

I recently read a quote from the great Fred Rogers, of the *Mr. Roger's*, television show that illustrates this point. He said that when he was a child, and he saw, or heard news of tragedy and death, it would upset him, until his mom told him *"Always look for the helpers."* What amazing advice. He spent most of his life doing just that: looking for the helpers and becoming one himself.

The point I'm trying to drive home here is that no matter how dark and tragic our story seems, we get to *choose* the story we want to write about it. If something as destructive and horrible as *war* has two sides to the Story Axe, so do all stories, including *yours*.

So the next time tragedy comes into *your* story, how will you write it? Will it be one of suffering and defeat? Or will you find a way to make it a story about Courage, Compassion, and our shared Humanity?

Why Stories?

Throughout this book, I've been telling you stories: all kinds of stories. There are at least a couple of reasons why. One, stories are engaging, if well told, and I hope mine have been. They grab and hold our attention. Two, stories convey meaning. The best stories do this without trying to do it. I mean they don't stop during the telling to *tell* you what the meaning is, like they did in the old Scooby Doo episodes: *"The moral of the story is that you shouldn't commit crimes in an old castle when the hippy van full of meddling kids are driving through the county!" "Also, make sure there aren't Scooby Snacks in your castle kitchen when you try to scare granny off of her property so you can put up condos. Just sayin'."*

Good stories have meaning in their bones. All good stories do, even when the writer doesn't realize it. In fact, it's always better for the story, the reader, and the meaning, if the author is completely oblivious to the underlying truth of the story, at least until after it's written. Otherwise, you get a Scooby story, which might be cute, but is devoid of any real power to teach, or move people to act.

Humans love stories
We just do.

Our minds tell us stories all day long, and even when we're asleep. We are essentially storytelling monkeys, with less hair. Well, some of you have less hair; I'm pretty hairy. I hate bananas, though. Just in case you were wondering if I was going to swing down out of a tree or something.

Humans developed the ability to tell stories so long ago in our evolution, that the origin is lost to us. This was probably a Monkey Brain development, when we started to distinguish the past, from the present. With that ability to remember past events, and dangers, our ancestors were able to construct mental—if not verbal—stories about those events, and bring them to mind when confronted with similar situations in the present.

This helped them to avoid dangers, like king cobras, lions, tigers, and bears, not to mention stampeding wildebeests. And if you've ever been run over by a bunch of pissed off wildebeests, you know it's something to avoid.

The Legend of Cousin Eddie and the Wildebeests
Our ape ancestor—let's call him Clark—probably sat in a tree, a couple million years ago, watching a not-yet-stampeding herd of wildebeests and remembered a story about his cousin Eddie (not

the one from *National Lampoon's Christmas Vacation* standing in his bathrobe emptying his camper toilet into the storm drain while smoking a cigar, just a monkey version of the same guy, well, a *more monkeyesque* version anyway) was messing around on the savanna one day when he inadvertently, on purpose, kicked a wildebeest in the scrotum, for fun — because that's what cousin Eddie type, monkey ancestors would do — and occasioned the entire herd to run rampant, leaving Eddie lying in a pile of bones, blood, and wildebeest shit.

This simple, if amusing, monkey story helped to keep Clark alive since it reminded him *not* to kick wild herding animals in the balls. That's awesome for us, because he's our grandfather. He passed down that storytelling ability to us, and now we can avoid being stampeded by wild beasts on the savanna and sneak out the back when Cousin Eddie arrives uninvited for Christmas dinner.

It's a handy tool to have, our Story Axe.

And a powerful one, because most of the stories we tell ourselves are very negative, indeed. Sometimes they're short stories, like "*I dropped my keys on the floor; I'm so stupid*:" mere statements of so-called fact, based on silly mistakes we make. I've called myself stupid for dropping my keys on the floor so many times that I can't even begin to count. If I *did* count them I'd be depressed as hell. But which is more stupid? Dropping your keys on the floor, or calling yourself stupid for doing it?

Of course, most of our negative stories aren't quite so silly, or so banal. They are longer, darker tales of tragedy, like "*I'm a Failure. I'm worthless, because I lost my job, and I'm never going to succeed because I'm not smart enough to learn a new trade or skill.*" And it continues, like a fuckin' soap opera, for decades, complete with the pathetic plots, bad acting, bad lighting, and the obligatory, wrong-side-of-the-tracks character in a leather jacket who is in love with the rich blonde chick who everyone loves, but she or he ends up with fuckin' amnesia — a condition so rare in real life, but apparently rampant in daytime TV — and they forget each other exists, and one of them almost dies, and then they finally figure out the '*who am I*' question and get married, and the pictures of the fictional event end up on magazine covers in every grocery store in the free world.

Who the hell wants to be in a story like that? Not me. I think I'd rather be weed-whipping marsh grass with Mr. No-Shoulders to be honest.

But we don't *have* to live pathetic, soap-opera stories. We don't have to go through life in a tragic tale of amnesia-ridden love and fake marriages. We also don't have to wade in water with poisonous snakes. There are TWO blades to every Story Axe! We can flip the axe around!

We can just rewrite the entire story!

FEAR AND EXCITEMENT: LIZARD BRAIN EXPERIENCE

Are You Experienced?

Months ago I interviewed a friend of mine, Jamie Rautenberg, for a YouTube series that I called, *Second Breakfast with Steve*. Jamie is a licensed psychotherapist, a holistic intuitive counselor, and general bad ass—if laughing, giggling, and being a Zen Mistress is bad ass, and I suppose it is. During our conversation, we landed on the topic of Fear—of course—and she said something that knocked me right out.

"Fear is just an experience. In fact, the physical symptoms are exactly the same as *excitement*."

"Wow!" I was shocked, but not completely. Something about it immediately made sense. It just *felt* like the truth. "Yeah, YEAH! I think you're right!"

Fear is an experience: like every other one.

Yeah, that's what I said. It's just an experience.

It is a sensation deep in our Lizard Brain, quickening the heart, racing blood to our core, to our legs, to our arms: prepping us for danger.

Will we fly?

Or will we fight?

But like Jamie said, Fear isn't the only thing that is experienced in this way: so is excitement.

Yes, in the Land of the Lizard, Fear is indistinguishable from excitement, and pain can feel like pleasure.

Think about it for a moment.

What's something you have a known Fear of doing?

Skydiving? Handling snakes? Public speaking? Think of something.

Then think of something that *you* do that some friend of yours thinks is terrifying?

There are people who bungie jump off of insanely tall bridges! Why do they do it? Aren't they scared shitless? Certainly seems like they should be. I wouldn't do it. I don't trust that cord to snap my big ass back up again before hitting the bottom of the river and smashing my brains out on a rock. But maybe you've done it? Or someone you know?

Maybe you've done zip lining? Looks pretty scary to me, though I would probably try that one.

Riding Serpents

Imagine you're 12 years old, again unless you *are* 12 years old. In which case just imagine yourself.

You're staring up at a massive green serpent, twisting and roaring through a forest, diving over a raging river. The sounds of a hundred people screaming are beating in your ears.

Would you join them on the serpent?

When I was 12, our church took a field trip to the amusement park, Busch Gardens Old Country in Williamsburg, Virginia. It was a youth group trip. There were about six of us kids going and my parents, the ministers were driving us up in the church van.

One of the topics on the way up was the awesome rides we were going to experience while there. Several of our favorites were bandied about until Tim Baggly yelled out:

"I want to ride the Loch Ness Monster!"

Tim was a kid with a lot of struggles in life, not the least of which was the teasing he got from the rest of us. Tim was physically and partially mentally disabled. I don't know what his specific condition was. All I know is that he struggled with them, and we didn't make it easier for him. It's not something I'm at all proud to admit. But that was the reality.

When Tim blurted out that he wanted to ride the biggest,

scariest roller coaster in the park, the dreaded Loch Ness Monster, there was only one response that my brother Dave and I could make:

"Yeah! We're definitely gonna do that!"

As soon as the words left my mouth, I started to shake inside. Fear rose in my Lizard Brain and I could feel it in my guts. I'm sure Dave felt it too, as he agreed with me, "Yeah! Definitely!"

My father continued to drive down the road, focused on his destination. Internally he was thinking, "*I hope they are just bluffing.*"

My dad had a severe Fear of rollercoasters, something he obtained as a young kid when his sister, Grace, took him to Coney Island back in the 40s. Grace was absolutely Fearless. She was the 'fun' aunt, the one that was always up for whatever adventure was at hand. And she dragged her little brother on the biggest, oldest, rickety wooden coaster at Coney Island. And that cured him of roller coasters for the next few decades.

In fact, he had such a Fear of them that he imparted it to his three sons. Thanks to his reluctance to ride the coasters, we had been infected with the same Fear and it had only been recently that Dave and I had attempted to ride even the most innocuous of the genre: the sleepy Scooby Doo roller coaster in the kids' section of Busch Gardens. I think the highest hill is about 12 feet off the ground or something: pretty pathetic as coasters go.

My dad, unbeknownst to us, was very much afraid that we might actually go through with our attempt to ride the big bad monster, so he hatched a devious plan.

When we entered the park, he ordered us to follow him. We did, not knowing where he was leading. He was moving at a brisk pace. We trotted along through the Renaissance themed part of Olde England at the front of the park until we reached Scotland.

My father stopped in his tracks.

We were standing at the entrance to the Loch Ness Monster.

"Well, here it is guys!" my dad said with as innocent a voice as he could muster. He was attempting to call our bluff; no doubt about it, that's what he was doing. I suddenly realized what he was up to. He figured that if he sprang it on us right then and there, we would break and we'd never find the courage to do it later in the day.

"If you're going to ride it, now's the best time of the day, before it gets too crowded!" he explained.

This was true, of course: very sound logic, and irrefutable.

Dave and I looked at each other, the Fear building in our stomachs again. We didn't actually say anything; we just stared at each other. I think he raised his eyebrows or something to ask, *"Are we really gonna do this?"*

I raised mine to say, *"Hell if I know!"*

But there was one kink in my father's brilliant plan. The Wild Card.

"Hey guys! Let's go!" Tim yelled. Tim was shuffling into the entrance, looking back with a smile on his face, and a questioning look that said, *"What are y'all waiting for?"*

There wasn't a hint of Fear in his eyes: not even a twitch of it.

I looked back at Dave.

He looked at me, and raised his eyebrows again, and grimaced a questioning smile to say, *"Dude, if we don't do this, we're never, ever gonna live it down."* If Tim wasn't afraid—the kid we made fun of all the time—then there was simply *no way* that we could back down. Not then.

And this was what my father had not anticipated: that Tim would *shame* us into facing our Fears. But that's exactly what happened. Shame—the Fear of Criticism, Loss of Status—is one powerful bastard, and not for the last time in my life, one Fear trumped another.

Dave and I reluctantly walked to the line which wasn't very long at all. That was a saving grace because we didn't have time to think about it too much. Tim was practically jumping up and down with excitement for the coming experience. Dave and I were scared shitless. My hands were cold and sweaty and Dave wouldn't stop talking. He went on and on and on. I don't even remember what he was talking about; it was too long ago. But I'm pretty sure I had no clue even then. My mind was on our impending doom.

We got nearer and nearer to the embarking point. The sound of the Monster was deafening as it roared over the tracks, people screaming in agony and Fear.

Finally, it was our turn. Dave and I got into a car near the middle of the coaster. That seemed like the safest place—not at the front where you would have to see everything that was coming at us, and not at the back, exposed to some unknown danger from behind.

Nessie slid out of the station, like a giant Mr. No-Shoulders. My stomach was in my throat.

The first part of the ride was fine. We glided through a peaceful forest on a slight downhill grade. But then we headed up. The Monster was dragged up the enormous hill by a massive chain under the track, *CLICK CLACK CLICK CLACK CLICK CLACK*, up we went, higher and higher.

Then we hit the top, went over a slight downward hill, and began to glide again, slowly picking up speed as we turned around the station, over it actually, headed through the tops of very tall Southern White Pines.

Then we were there.

The drop was ahead. We could see it as we made a turn to the right.

Down we went. Everyone else was screaming.

Dave and I were silent with Fear.

The bottom of the world fell out from under us, and we plunged towards the raging river at the bottom of the canyon. Our stomachs were in our throats. Our hearts were pounding in our ears.

Five seconds later...

We were roller coaster *addicts*.

The Fear we had experienced all the way to Virginia in the van, even up to the entrance to the ride, had been suddenly transformed into Excitement and Exhilaration.

We got on that Monster as characters in *one* story: Fear.

We got off minutes later as heroes in a *new* one: Excitement.

Thank you, Timmy Baggley, wherever you are, for the push over that hill.

And that is how simple it is to overcome Fear, my friend. You simply have to rewrite the story you tell around it. The sensations of Fear and Excitement feel the same, absolutely the same. The only difference, *the only one*, is the story we tell ourselves about that experience. Change the story, change everything. Change the story and you can End Fear Itself.

YOUR INNER RED RIDING HOOD: A BASKET OF VICTIMHOOD

What kind of story are you telling right now?

What tale do you weave about yourself, about your life, your personality, your abilities, your talents?

Is it a positive, uplifting story? Or is it like most of us, decidedly negative?

Are you Little Red Riding Hood? Hansel or Gretel? Are you the victim in the story?

If you're like me, and most people, the answer is probably yes, in at least one of your stories. We've already covered the theory behind this and why most of us tell such shitty stories about ourselves and beat ourselves up over the silliest things. Now it's time to do something to change that. *It's time to write the victim out.*

A couple years ago, I read a handful of books on positive psychology. One that stood out to me was by Jim Loehr: *The Power of Story*. Loehr has developed a technique, or exercise, that I really love and employed myself to help me deal with a lot of negative issues and emotions that I was experiencing. And it involves storytelling. I've borrowed what I think are the best ideas from Loehr's technique, as well as from Tim Ebl's book, *Demons in the Cellar*, and combined them with a few of my own ideas to create a hybrid technique which produces amazing results.

Dropping the Basket of Victimhood

This is how it works: the first step in rewriting our personal story.

1. **Assemble Your Materials:** Take out your journal, a legal pad, or several sheets of paper. You can do this on the computer as well, but I think it works better if you physically write it out. Psychologists have recently discovered that we learn more effectively if we write things out by the hand, than if we type it. Both methods work but handwriting is more effective.

2. **Write Out Your Story:** Write it in 3rd person. In other

words, write it as if you were telling someone *else's* story. For example: *"Steve is a loser. He never finishes anything he starts. He's always broke and never succeeds financially, despite having shitloads of talent and education."*

- Write as *fast as you can*. I don't mean every detail. We're not trying to write a book, just a brief summary. It's a highlights reel, if you will: the main events, emotions, people in your life, and your feelings about them. Don't stop to edit, spellcheck, think about what you've written, or analyze it. Just FEEL it, and go, go, go! Dump it all out as fast as you possibly can! You should be able to do this in less than 30 minutes.

- **Let the Toxins Out**: Dr. Loehr suggests that you write the version of your story that you actually tell yourself, every day: your *victim* story, the one where you point out all the negative things that have happened to you, your Fears, your failures, your hates, the things that are wrong with you (too fat, too skinny, too stupid, too slow, too old, too ugly, you get the picture), your angst, your depression, your melancholy, the people who have wronged you and what you want to do to them. All the things that hold you back from doing what you really want to do in life. DO NOT HOLD BACK. Do not censor it; let it all out! Consider the page to be your punching bag, your handkerchief, the beer for all your tears. No one is going to see this, unless you want to show it to someone, and I doubt you will. Mine was toxic as hell and I bet yours will be, too.

3. **Take a Break**: DO NOT READ THE STORY! You need time away from it. Take a nap, a walk around the block, go jogging, swimming, or gardening. Let that story sit for at least 24 hours. I think it's important to do this. You're gonna read it, but it's best to let it rest.

4. **Meditate:** After 24 hours, or more, come back to what you've written. Maybe meditate first to help clear the mind, or pray, or do whatever you do to calm your mind.

5. **Read Your Story:** Read it out loud, if possible, to yourself.

Listen to it. Notice any emotions that come up as you read. Don't do anything about them; just notice them.

6. **Dig for Truth:** Now, go back through the story, line by line. As much as possible, approach it from an objective mindset, as if you were reading a friend's story. Ask yourself, about each and every negative thing within it, the following questions:

- Is this true? Is it factually true?

- Do I really *believe* it to be true?

- What would the people closest to me think about what I've said about myself? *Is* this what they think about me?

Go through this process for the entire story, for each and every negative statement you've written. Make notes. Circle or highlight things that stand out as false. Maybe highlight any true statements, as well, possibly with a different color.

What I think you're going to find, is that the vast majority of the negative things you say about yourself is complete bullshit. Mine was almost all bullshit. Sure, there were some factual elements in there: things that actually happened to me. But the story I had written *around* it, especially the nasty things I said about myself, were all bullshit.

There is something quite liberating to writing the toxins out, dumping all of that negativity onto the page, onto the Forest floor, like so much mental diarrhea. But that kind of crap is much better outside of the mind, than in it, and writing it down is the best way I know of kicking it to the curb. So let's move on to the next step: our new story.

BE THE WOODSMAN: FROM VICTIM TO HERO

"There is no great writing, only great rewriting." —Louis Brandeis, Supreme Court Justice

Most of the stuff I've ever written was pretty messy and sometimes downright shitty as it stood in the first draft. First drafts are supposed to suck. They don't always suck, but most of the time they do. The key to writing is to just *get it out* of your head and onto the page. It's not the version you want to publish, unless you want to run all your readers away.

The magic of writing usually comes in the subsequent drafts; the *rewriting* as Justice Brandeis mentioned. So why should it be any different with the stories we tell about our lives? I mean, if Stephen King gets to rewrite *his* stories, why can't we rewrite *ours*? The answer, of course, is that we *can*!

"But what happened is what happened!" you say.

"Oh hell no it ain't!" I shout back at you.

There is no such thing as objective reality.

Reality is absolutely what you want to make of it: 100%.

That doesn't mean that things don't happen *to you*. They do. But the truth is that only *you* assign *meaning* to those events. Only you.

You are a storywriter.

You are the author of your own life because you create a story around everything that ever happens to you, every thing you do, every choice you make. You do this every waking hour of your life, and probably a lot of the sleeping hours, too.

Your story, the story you tell inside your own head, *is your reality*.

Let me repeat it: Your story *IS YOUR REALITY*.

There is no other reality for you.

The *fastest* way to End Fear Itself is to just rewrite the story you tell about it.

After you've written out and analyzed your toxic story, you can rewrite it with a positive slant. And that's what you're getting ready to do, right now!

Be the Hero, not the Victim!

It's time to stop playing the victim in your own life's story. You are a badass! You are the hero! And your story should be one with lots of deep, dark Forests, wolves, lions, tigers, and fuckin' bears but *they* should be dinner, not YOU! You're the hunter, the woodsman with a double-bladed axe. Sure, you could cut your toe off with the wrong side of it if you're not careful but those days are over! It's time to flip that thing over and swing away! Let's hack up that victim story and rewrite it as a heroic comedy.

Here's how you do it:

1. **Review Your Victim Version:** After you've had a chance to let your negative story sit for a couple of days, at least, go back to it again and view it from a detached point of view.

2. **Rethink the Story:** Now we're going to start changing the nature of your story. Instead of seeing yourself as the victim headed for disaster, tragic death and failure, start thinking about it as the story of an epic struggle against overwhelming odds in which you triumph in the end. Yes, we'll put a temporary ending on it, but one of success.

3. **Rewrite It!:** This time, write it in 1st person perspective! For example: "*I am the greatest writer in history! Despite demons, Balrogs, orcs, and dragons, as well as my own Fear of Inadequacy, I will prevail! My book,* The End of Fear Itself, *is going to sell millions of copies, end war, eradicate poverty and greed, and usher in a Utopia on Earth!*" Now, THAT'S a story worth reading!

    -   Make sure to emphasize the positive things that *actually* happened in the story: your friends or family who were there for you, the times you were successful, the inner strength you displayed through overwhelming odds. Imagine yourself as Frodo or Rocky or Princess Leia, or some other heroic movie character. You are the champion of your own story!

4. **Write a Happy Ending:** And when you come to the present circumstances in your story, project it into the future. It doesn't have to be a long time into the future, a few months, or a year or so is fine. Just so long as during that period you accomplish something major in your life that you are working toward, or preparing to work toward. Choose one of your current goals and write an ending that features you

as the Master of the Universe!

5. **Take Another Break:** Let the story sit for another day or so, then read it back to yourself, out loud. How does it feel? A bit cheesy? Probably, but that's okay. If you keep working on your Afformations©, over time you'll start to believe this new story. It's definitely a better way to look at life than as a victim. Being a victim just sucks. Sure, that story served the *old* you, the one that was in Fear of Failure, of Success, of everything, but not the *new* you, the courageous, heroic badass that you really are.

6. **Come Back to Your Story:** Read this story to yourself once a day for at least a month. I like to do it in the morning before everyone else gets up. Then, come back to it any time you start to feel that Riding Hood mentality creeping back in.

In the next section, we'll take our new heroic mentality back out into that dark forest and clean up the debris of our Tree of Fear: the random, *windfall* fruits of that poisonous tree. Get your rake! It's time to clean up the forest floor.

Raking Up the Forest Floor: Roots and Branches, Twigs and Dust

Once you've yanked out the Seed of Inadequacy and applied the Axes of Afformations©, Forgiveness, and Storytelling to the trunk of known Fears you'll find that most of the Fears you used to think were so important have simply fallen away. At the very least, they will have significantly less power in your life. But just in case there's some lingering detritus lying around in the Forest of your mind, we'll get out our rakes and sweep them all away, maybe toss them into a compost bin to turn them into useful soil.

There are a handful of special rakes for this job. We'll start with the ancient art of Meditation.

MEDITATION: THE RAKE OF ZEN AND TAO

"I have lived with several Zen masters -- all of them cats." —Eckhart Tolle, Master of Now, and apparently, also a cat

Even once we deal with all of our root and trunk Fears, and have excavated the Seed of Inadequacy, there are still sometimes lingering projected Fears and, of course, an occasional new one which may pop up. Ending Fear Itself doesn't mean getting rid of *all* Fear; it just means that we've broken the hold it had on us and turned it into a *verb*. We've moved from *having Fear* to fear*ing*. So we need some methods to rake up all of those windfall Fruits and clean up the forest floor every once in a while when a new Fear pops up or blows into our life. One of the best ways to deal with these is through some form of meditation.

A Zen for the Unbendy: Meditation 101

For many years, I've struggled with meditation. Pretty much, I suck at it. Or at least I thought I did. That's just because I was doing it wrong. Actually, I was just *thinking* about it in the wrong way and this is pretty common. I'll try to dispel a couple of pervasive myths about meditation that might be stumbling blocks for you as they were for me.

"I don't know the right way to meditate!"

I spent many years trying to find the *best* way to meditate. I tried staring at candles, focusing on my breath, listening to *Woo Woo* Zen masters talk me through walks along imaginary beaches, ancient forests, and bingo parlors full of blue-haired grannies. But none of them seemed to work. I couldn't focus for more than a few seconds on any of it without my brain wandering off to the bar next door to the Bingo Bonanza. [I made up the bingo meditation. It just popped into my head, so I figured I'd leave it. I've never actually *been* in a bingo parlor. I'm making this shit up as I go.]

I just couldn't focus. I was sure I was really screwing it up royally. So then, I would mentally self-flaggelate to punish myself for being a crappy meditator. I did this until I read somewhere that I really shouldn't beat myself up. Instead, I should just keep bringing my attention back to my candle, or Ethel's blue hair, or the *B,14* square on my bingo card. But it just didn't seem to work. I couldn't do it. I'm *still* not any good at it.

Place Your Right Hand on Blue, Left Foot on Yellow

You're probably starting to wonder if I ever figured out how to meditate?

Well, I did, but only after realizing that the other thing I was concerned about wasn't necessary, either: sitting in a Lotus position. I tried it and failed miserably. I don't bend. I'm un-bendy, like a tree, or a steel beam. I don't sit down; I kind of just *flop* down in my chair or on the bed. So the whole Zen Master Pretzel Position was out! Hell no. It was too much playing Twister with clothes on sans baby oil. So I just sat in a chair and stared at *B, 14,* while Ethel reattached her teeth next to me and showed me photos of her grandkids.

Then entered the Laughing German Buddha from England: Eckhart Tolle

I was watching a video on YouTube one day in which this funny little guy with a German accent, Eckhart Tolle, was talking about meditation and the myths and misunderstandings about it. He introduced an idea that *anyone* can do! He calls it Mini Meditation.

Instead of worrying about finding a quiet spot with no distractions—which is basically impossible in our modern homes— you can meditate *anywhere* and at *anytime*.

Here's how it works:

1. For as little as 5 to 10 seconds—yes, that's what I said, seconds—just focus your full attention on whatever you're doing in the moment.

2. Don't make this difficult. You can focus on washing your hands, the feel of your feet on the floor as you walk around the house, the feeling and sound of your fingers as they type on your laptop. It doesn't matter. Anything.

3. That's it! You're done! I told you it was simple.

4. Repeat. Do this whenever you think to do it. Set up an alarm on your phone to remind you to do it throughout the day. The more often you do it, the more often you will *remember* to do it.

5. You've just meditated. Congratulations!

To apply this to your remaining Fears, or fearing that comes up at any time, you can do the following things:

Focus

I think the first step in dealing with any Fear is to focus our conscious attention upon it. Turn it into a Mini Meditation. We have to realize what's going on when it happens. This doesn't mean that we can always stop ourselves from slipping into a negative state of mind; that takes a lot of practice. It doesn't always stop the emotions but sometimes we can slow it down and keep from making our little brain spin into a complete Whirlpool of Piss.

Put on the Brakes

The next step in a very long process is to slow down the negative spin by focusing on it even more. At first, this will feel more like taking some of the wind out of the event. As you say to yourself, *"Self, you're losing control of your emotions. This is just a reaction to a Fear that you have about 'fill in blank'."* Once you say this, you'll feel the whirlpool start to slow down. It won't stop, not the first time you do this. But eventually, you'll get to the point where it stops and you can start rebuilding your positive energy. This takes a long time and a lot of practice to do. I'm still working on it, but one day I *will* master it! And so will you!

Be Like Barney: Do Some Bud-nippin

Once we manage to bring some attention to a Fear, then we can slowly begin to *nip it in the bud*, as Barney Fife used to say on the Andy Griffith Show. This is where we begin to master our minds. Bud-nippin is a very Zen art. I am happy to say that I have managed to stop a couple of whirlpools before they spun out of control. It's quite satisfying when you can manage it. I've only done it a couple of times, but I know it can be done, and that's most of the battle. Once you've been able to slow down and bring your emotions to a halt a few times, start focusing on trying to feel them when they begin to spin, before they are out of control, and nip them in the bud.

If you can catch that first or second negative thought before it has time to gather friends and become a gang, you can stop the entire process before it becomes a whirlpool. You have to develop a big red STOP sign in your brain that you can throw up in your mind's eye, whenever a negative thought enters the brain. This is the goal. The ultimate goal would be to eliminate all negative thoughts but I don't think that's actually possible. I've never even heard a Zen master claim such powers. Maybe some have achieved it but, if so, they've kept quiet about it.

While these three techniques seem simple, and they are, they are very difficult to master. It takes time and focus to do it. You will fail many more times than you succeed. Just don't give up trying. When whirlpools come and take you over just let them ride out and dissipate. Then ask yourself, *"Why am I able to stop my negative thoughts and turn them into positive ones?"* This is an Afformation.© Say it out loud to yourself so your brain registers it subconsciously. It works. You won't remember to do it all the time, but the more you do it the more often you will remember to do it. It's like learning anything else; it takes time and repetition.

Eventually, you'll get to the point where your conscious focus will kick in every time you go into a negative spin. And then the spins won't last as long and you probably won't do as much damage to your relationships, including the one you have with yourself. Then, one day, you'll manage to catch the spin before it goes out of control and stop it dead in its tracks!

Once you begin to master them, you can also begin to see the humor in them.

HUMOR: LAUGHING IN THE FOREST OF FEAR

"When you recognize drama as drama, it becomes, also, funny." — Eckhart Tolle

"Tragedy is when I have a hangnail. Comedy is when you accidentally walk into an open sewer and die." — Mel Brooks, comedian, film-maker, and master of sarcasm

Where did you meet your significant other's parents?

I met Paysh's family in the morgue.

Top *that one*!

Think about that one for a second. And I'm *not* making this up to impress you, or *depress* you either. It's simply a fact.

Can you think of a more awkward way to 'meet the parents?'

I doubt it.

The Story

When Patience and I had just started dating, she called me one morning on her way to work, in tears, the kind that comes with difficulty in breathing.

"Tony, my brother-in-law, was killed in an accident last night."

"Oh my god," I said, "No!"

I was instantly sad myself though I'd never met him. I hadn't met *anyone* in the family, yet, but I knew from Paysh's description that Tony was a person I was looking forward to knowing.

"I'm supposed to go down to Hastings!" she said, in between sobs, "but I don't think I can drive right now."

"*I'll* drive you!" I said without even thinking. It was simply the only thing I could do for her at that moment, so I said it without even thinking about the ramifications.

So, I drove my new girlfriend to the morgue.

And that's where I met every adult in the Felt clan. All of them, including her poor sister, Heidi, who had just lost her husband. Talk about surreal. I did my best to just be a wallflower. I felt very much like I was invading a private space, like watching a stranger take a shower or something. And my emotions and feelings had nothing to do with the family's words or actions toward me, far from it. In fact, they did their best to be gracious and thanked me for driving Paysh down and all that, but this was definitely *not* the place any of us would have chosen to meet.

Who would?

But I'm not telling this story just to tell you how awkward my 'meet the parents' experience was. I want to talk about the meaning of life, and how we can make it as good as it can be.

I want to talk about the relationship between Tragedy and Comedy.

Most people think that the two things are mutually exclusive. I do not. I tend to agree with the great Mel Brooks; tragedy and comedy depend entirely upon one's perspective. And one's perspective changes over time.

When tragedy strikes, as it did when Tony died, it's very difficult to remember the funny stuff for a while. The pain is too great, and the closer you are to the tragedy—as Mel Brooks pointed out—the harder it is to bridge the gap from *tragedy* to *comedy*. A hangnail can be a bitch, man.

From Tragedy to Comedy: Narrowing the Gap

I think that the key to life—and I do mean the **main key**—is to shorten the gap between tragedy and comedy till it's almost non-existent. I mean *SQUEEZE* that fucker till it POPS!

If we can learn to laugh at *anything*, to find the comedy in all situations, if we can do it almost instantaneously, then we will be laughing Buddhas. What is to be happy, to be joyful, other than that ability? Life is chock full of tragic events, personal ones, family ones, human ones. Are we to go around weeping and lamenting them constantly?

Hell no! That would be a very sad existence indeed.

I tell people, often, that when I die, if I swoop down over the funeral and see a bunch of people weeping, I'm gonna come back from the dead and kick their ass! I want to see a party the likes of which has never been thrown before! I want to see fire, and booze, and BBQ, and axe-throwing, and laughter, or I'm gonna become a poltergeist and run them all out of my yard!

I think that we take life too seriously.

Why do we do that?

I think we do it simply because our parents told us that life was something to be serious about! Look around you, almost everyone is overly serious. Work is serious, life is a serious struggle to stave off death, to get 'ahead' whatever that means. Ahead of what? Death? Disease? Hunger? Cold?

What are we trying to get ahead of?

Can we get ahead of it? I think not. Those things just *are*. Maybe. Maybe they're not.

The late great philosopher, Alan Watts, used to say that life wasn't serious at all. It might be sincere, but never serious. For Watts, the purpose of life was simply to live it, much the same as to dance. "What is the purpose of dancing?" Watts would ask, then answer,

"To dance!" It's not to reach a certain place on the floor. The same goes for music. If reaching the final cadence and chord were the point, all symphonies, or big-hair rock power ballads would contain only one chord! But they don't. Because the point is to dance; the point is to let the music wash over you. It isn't to get to the end.

Humor as Meditation

If we stop taking our Fears so seriously they cease to bother us, or exist at all. The way I do this, when I do it, is to step back like an observer and just watch my Fear.

Let's take the Fear of Being Wrong, for instance. I know I have this Fear. Sometimes I see it creep up on me; I actually notice it happening. This is like stepping out of the play and becoming someone in the audience of a comedy. When I do that, I can be a bit more detached from my Fear. It becomes something outside of myself that I can watch.

From that perspective I can see more clearly the absurdity of my Fears, my actions, my thoughts. I suddenly realize just how ridiculous they are, even if just for an instant. At first, this may be all we can accomplish. It's a mini-meditation. We are meditating on our own Fears, using them as a point of concentration so we can laugh at them.

If you can get to the point where you laugh at one of your Fears you will begin to feel a great lifting inside you. It's as if you had been on a long hike through the forest with a heavy backpack and you stopped for a break and took it off. The feeling you get from laughing at your own Fears is similar. The more you are able to do it, the lighter you will feel.

And you don't have to wait around for one of your Fears to rear it's ugly head. You can just bring up one of them when you're in a *good* mood and make fun it it! This is actually one of the most powerful types of meditation and it's been around for a very long time. Ancient Buddhist monks have been practicing laughing meditation for millennia.

I once took a class at East Carolina University with a religious studies professor, Calvin Mercer, who had us all sit around the room, some on the floor, some on sofas and chairs. Then he told us that for the next ten minutes, a full ten minutes, we were all going to laugh out loud.

Yeah, I know, it sounds weird as hell. And it is. But it's also effective.

For ten minutes, we laughed. And we laughed. At first, we had to force the laughter, because there's nothing really to laugh about, or at least that's what I thought. But after a minute or two, we were all laughing at the absurdity of laughing about nothing and then the whole thing became hysterical in and of itself.

When the ten minutes were up, my mind, spirit, and body were floating. There was a huge relief and release of negative energy and influx of positive to replace it.

Laughing in the Forest of Fear: Mini Meditation with a Chuckle

We can use laughter as a form of Mini Meditation to dispel the negative energy of Fear when it arises.

Laughing at one of our Fears won't give you quite the high you get from laughing at nothing for ten minutes, but it *will* give you a boost and help you to get past that particular Fear. Eventually, the more you laugh at them the faster your Fears retreat. The more you laugh at anything will do this.

Find things to laugh at during your day.

What about the guy who cut you off in traffic?

Just think to yourself for a second, *"Gotta to get to the gym!"* and imagine that's what he's thinking as he races past you down the road.

This is what Paysh, Duke, and I say every time we see someone racing down the road as if life were serious as hell. One of us, usually Duke, will yell out, *"Gotta get to the gym!!!"* Then we chuckle and shake our heads. It's not a fully on belly laugh, just a few chuckles at the other driver's expense. But it keeps us from flying into a rage about inconsiderate drivers on the road and ruining our day.

If you're faced with a Fear and can bring enough realization upon it to allow yourself to step out into the audience for a moment, notice just how absurd your Fear is. How comical. And laugh. Even if it's just a little chuckle and shake of your head it will work wonders towards your goal of being Fear free.

LAUGH people! Life isn't serious. It simply isn't. It might be *sincere*, but never fuckin' serious. It's a game, a play. Let's make it a comedy, and stop thrashing around like we're in the middle of Macbeth or Hamlet. Personally, I think it's a comedy. I didn't always think that way but I'm becoming more and more convinced that it is. Stop taking yourself and your Fears so seriously. Laugh at them and be free.

Remember, we can choose how we want to live our lives. No one else writes our story; it's ours alone to write. It is our most potent power. Will it be a tragedy? Or will it be a comedy? I vote for comedy.

I'm not saying we have to laugh at *all* of our Fears or every tragic situation that we find ourselves in. Sometimes there is real loss, like the Felt family experienced when Tony was killed. Sometimes it's not yet time to laugh. But we can still deal with our Fear of Loss. Once the grief or anger passes, we can focus not on what we've lost, but on what we've gained.

FLIPPING THE FEAR OF LOSS: WHAT DO I GAIN?

Sometimes our loss is so great, that it's nearly impossible to focus on anything positive. But the sooner we can do that, the better.

Even in the case of loss due to death, we can find things we've gained.

When someone we care about dies, our Fear of Loss shifts. We no longer fear losing them; they're already gone. What we fear is dealing with the hole they left behind. We fear the pain of not having them around anymore: that they're gone forever. But they're not.

Tony is still very much alive, even if he's not physically present. He lives on, every day, in the hearts of his children, his widow, his family, and his friends. And I know that statement can sound like a platitude, a catch-phrase we all use in situations of death and tragedy. But in Tony's case, it's just a fact.

By all accounts, Tony was one of the funniest men on Earth: full of life, laughter, compassion, loyalty, and all the other traits of a great man. I am actually shedding tears as I write this, and I never met him. But I *feel* that I have. In fact, I *have* met him. I talk with him, hear his stories, his jokes, even his laugh, through the stories his family tells of him. Not one family event goes by without several 'Tony Stories.' His life is an endless well of smiles and laughter. Is there anything better that one could say about us when we're 'gone' than that? I think not.

What did the Felt family gain from Tony? They gained years of memories, great ones, funny ones, and he left behind a beautiful family. The loss was great, but so was the gain.

Count the Gains

Not all loss is due to death, of course. We fear losing all kinds of things, silly things mostly.

One of the problems with the Fear of Loss is that we are uber-focused on what we might *lose*. We become so fixated on the things we might have to give up, like bacon, sugar, and ice cream — if we're trying to lose weight — that we lose sight of what we might actually *gain* from the change: better health and more energy, for instance.

The fixation on Loss and the Fear that comes with it is an extension of our proclivity towards negativity which stems from our Lizard Brain. Just because it's natural for us to Fear change and loss doesn't mean we have to keep doing it. Fear*ing* loss is one thing; having a *Fear* of Loss is another.

Instead of focusing on what we might *lose*, let's focus on what we might, and most likely would, *gain* from any situation. This tiny shift is really not so tiny and it isn't difficult to learn. We just have to apply the STOP sign we talked about earlier whenever the Fear of Loss pops up.

Once you realize that you are experiencing Fear of Loss:

1. STOP for a second and think to yourself, *"How likely am I to actually lose something here?"*

2.   Then ask, "*What might I gain from this change or experience?*" If it's a big change and not just a decision about where to go for dinner, then you might need to do a pro/con list. But don't give the cons too much attention, at least not more attention than you give the pros. Most of us tend to give the cons way too much credit and weight in our decision processes.

3.   Once you've made the list of pros and cons, take a look at it. Do the cons really outweigh the pros? Really? Maybe, in some cases, they might. But don't just look at the *number* of pros versus cons; look at the *weight* of each item.

For instance, let's say you're trying to decide whether or not to go into business for yourself, and leave your nine to five job. You have a list with an equal number of pros and cons, or maybe five more cons than pros. Should you abandon the idea? Not necessarily.

If you look at the relative importance of each thing on the list, are they equal? Is having free, crappy coffee in the break room, really more important than having more time to spend with your family? Is the illusion of safety at your old job really more important than the financial freedom that might come from building your own business? Or is it just the Fear of Loss holding you back from making a change?

Sometimes the losses are real and significant. These come to us in times of crisis: illness, accidents, even death to a loved one or friend. They're tough times, for sure. These are times when Fear can snowball if we don't get a grip on it. That's where the 4th step comes in.

4. What is the Lesson?

It's perfectly natural to feel loss and the Fear that comes with it in these situations. It's not necessary to stop all fearing from happening; it's not even possible. Fearing is natural. Having Fears is, too, but Fears aren't healthy in the long run. Let fearing take its course. But before fearing becomes a Fear, throw up the STOP sign and ask yourself one simple question: "*What positive lesson can I learn from this painful experience?*" This is one of the most important questions to learn and apply in our lives. Always be looking for the lessons to learn from your experiences, but *especially* from the negative ones. There is *always* something positive to learn. Always.

Maybe the lesson is simply that, *"I am suffering, but all suffering will pass."*

Or, *"I have survived many such things; I will walk through this one as well."*

It is important to remember that we have suffered before, that we have been afraid before and we survived it. It's easy when we're in the middle of a painful experience, a scary one, to forget just how many times we have been in such places and that we always found a way to come through them. We can do it again as many times as we need to.

This particular trick is one that I've used to come through some pretty tough shit in my life: death of friends and family, two divorces, business failures, job terminations, a house fire, depressions, foreclosure, repossessions, debt, rejections, and probably a bunch more that I can't remember. Even at my worst moments, deep inside of me, there was a tiny voice telling me, *"You've been through worse crap. You'll make it through this."*

And when that voice wasn't strong enough to bring me out on its own it was just strong enough to compel me to reach out for help. Because in the end, it is our connections to other people that really make life worth living. There are always people out there who care about us. Never forget to reach out to those around you. If they are true friends, and good family, then they *want* to be helpful. We all want to be needed and helpful, so accept help graciously whenever you can. You might be helping someone feel needed and important by allowing them to help you. This is a win-win for everyone.

Friends and family are immensely helpful when we're faced with the tough processes of life, and the Fears that come with them. We can reach out to our friends and family to help us keep on keeping on. You can also reach out to professionals: doctors, psychologists, psychiatrists, counselors, and coaches. A great coach is worth every penny. I wouldn't trade Bobby Kountz for anything.

Once you've given some thought to what you might *gain* by facing your Fears, you can add all those things to a long list of pluses you can be grateful for.

THE BROOM OF GRATITUDE: GOODBYE FEAR, HELLO HAPPY HELMET

One of the most popular tools for cleaning up Fear and it's nasty fruits is the Broom of Gratitude.

When I first began writing this book, this was one of my go-to cures. It still is, but it requires a preface.

Best for Clean-up and Daily Sprucing

There's a popular movement around gratitude that suggests it's the panacea for all our problems. I have been a proponent of it myself. And it is an essential tool to achieving happiness and fulfillment in life. However, it can sometimes obscure underlying Fears and negative experiences that we haven't really dealt with. This often comes across as *fake* gratitude, which doesn't do anyone any good.

Life coach, Philip McKernan, brought this point up recently and it got me to thinking. While he and I agree that gratitude is a very important tool in achieving happiness and well-being, if it is our *only* tool, it tends to overshadow some of the root digging and tree chopping that we need to do in order to really get to the crux of our problems. It simply isn't good enough to *say* you're grateful and happy; you have to do the work to actually *get* there. And some of that is more difficult than just focusing on what's *good* in your life.

That being said, part of the process of finding happiness and bringing about the End of Fear Itself, is to realize that we already have a lot of great things in our lives. Along with the other work of digging up those roots and hacking up stumps, one of the best things we can do to combat Fear is to start practicing gratitude.

"But only happy people have anything to be grateful for!" you say. That's what I thought, too, but it's incorrect. The inverse is the truth; **people who practice gratitude become happier**. Period.

Yes, happy people tend to practice gratitude more but it is the cause and effect that we have gotten wrong. We've turned them round the wrong way; gratitude *precedes* happiness, not the other way round. Once you're happy, you will be more grateful than ever, so it creates an awesome feedback loop. But gratitude comes first. This isn't a chicken and egg thing.

Where I Found the Magic Broom of Gratitude

I came across this idea, first, in a book by Jane McGonigal, *Reality is Broken*, in which she mentioned the work of Martin Seligman and other positive psychologists, and was stunned by the simplicity of the idea. So stunned, that it took me a year or more to realize that I really needed to *apply* the knowledge. It turns out, that just knowing where the broom *hangs*, isn't the same as sweeping with it. You have to actually *do it*, i.e., practice gratitude, in order to get the benefit of happiness.

Jane also mentioned an app in her book that helps to keep you on track when it comes to practicing gratitude, aptly named, **The Happier App**!

Happier App: The Broom Closet of Happiness

The free app—which you should look up and download—was developed by an awesome lady, Natalie Kogan. It's very simple to use. The layout is similar to Facebook. You are encouraged to post small moments of gratitude throughout your day and share them with your social media outlets: Facebook and Twitter, as well as people who follow you on Happier. You can then comment and 'smile' at other people's moments.

There are also 'courses' in gratitude, some of them free, that you can opt into that help to explain the core ideas of living a more grateful, happier life. Natalie's courses are the best, I think.

Trust me, it works.

You're probably thinking, "Yeah, whatever. You're just one of those 'naturally' happier people."

WRONG! If you want to know where my mind was a few years ago, just read my first blog post on stevebivans.com: *My Negative Life: a Positive Twist*, and you'll see the arc of my journey from a very negative space to where I am today: a happy man. And the Happier App played no small part in that transformation.

Sweeping the Forest Floor with Gratitude

Here's how you do gratitude:

1. Set a timer on your phone using HiFutureSelf, or your calendar app, to remind you to do this at least three times during the day. It should say something like, "Practice gratitude, NOW!"

2. When the timer goes off, stop what you're doing, unless you're driving or having sex or something important.

3. Think of 3 things you're grateful for. They can be anything from as small a thing as, *"I'm grateful for this car I'm driving or this person next to me,"* or as grand as, *"I'm grateful for the whole Universe and the pretty stars in the sky."*

4. If you are able, write these things down. You can write them on paper, in Evernote, on a chalkboard in your kitchen — something we do at our house, or open up Happier App and post them on there.

5. Thank people when you're out and about: at the store, the bank, the gym.

6. Join my friend, Chris Palmore's group, Gratitude Space, on Facebook!

7. Add some kindness to your gratitude: Pay it forward by buying coffee for the guy behind you in line, or giving a larger tip to your server at lunch. Be creative!

8. That's it!

Do practice gratitude. Start now, even if you haven't begun any of the other exercises in the book. It *does* make a difference. Don't skip all the other steps to bring down your Tree of Fear. You can't very well dig up the Seed of Inadequacy with a broom; it takes a shovel. But gratitude can help you get through the forest *to* the Tree, and give you courage to keep digging and chopping, until you have that damn Tree down and ground into sawdust.

Gratitude will be there as a natural result of all that work, in the end, when you are ready to plant a new Tree and transform that Forest into a garden of plenty.

Pruning the Fear of Process

Lopping off the limb of the Fear of Process is a tricky one, because the Fear Itself is so twisted and elusive. It's not a Fear of something concrete. Not that any of our Fears *are* concrete; they aren't. But Loss and Outcome are at least things we can *measure*. We had something and now we don't: 1 to 0. Outcome is the same way. We attempted something and we either failed or succeeded.

But Process is a longer event, a bunch of things we have to do, or go through in order to either lose or gain something. It's hard to point at the Process. It's much easier to point at the empty hole where something once was.

Since Process is so twisted and vaporous the cures for it are also a bit less solid.

That doesn't mean they don't *work*, just that they aren't simple 1, 2, 3 steps. They involve ideas like acceptance, focus, and meditation.

BE A SCARECROW: YOUR BRAIN IN THE NOW

"Oh I could tell you why
the ocean's near the shore.
I could think of things I'd never thunk before.
and then I'd sit, and think some more.
I would not be just a nothin'
my head all full of stuffin'
my heart all full of pain.
I would dance and be merry,
life would be a ding-a-derry

if I only had a brain." —Scarecrow, *The Wizard of Oz,* movie, 1939

How to Calm the Chaos

One way to deal with Chaos is to get a little more organized.

You don't have to become anal-retentive, just tidy up a bit in the brain. You don't really have to clean up your office, though that would be a good idea, too. Mostly you just need to clean out your Monkey Brain before it becomes an episode of Hoarders.

The best way to do this is to write all the crap in your brain down on an actual list. I call it a brain-dump. It helps eliminate brain-spin. If you let it go for too long, and then throw in some negative stimuli you get a *Whirlpool of Piss*; nobody wants that.

But lists themselves can be a distraction if we haven't made some connection to *time*. It's not just putting things on a list that's important. We also need to give an indication of *when* we're going to get around to doing the tasks or our mind will continue to worry about them.

Schedule a regular time of day, or a day each week to review your 'to do lists.' This helps keep you from worrying about all the stuff on there while you're working on other tasks.

Just Let Go and Let It Be

Clearing out the mind and cleaning up our living and working spaces is great, but the best cure for the Fear of Chaos—a disease we all suffer from—is to let it go.

The ancient Chinese philosophy of Taoism has some illustrative points on this topic. One might argue that the entire philosophy is based on the idea that we have no *control*, only influence. If you ever read the *Dao de Jing*, you'll find the metaphor of water is central to the entire idea of Dao.

The Dao (usually translated as the way, the Universe, everything) is like a flowing river. We are all in the river and can be in no other place. We can choose either to swim *with* the river or *against* it. Either way, we move down stream.

Much like my brother and I that night long ago in the ocean, if you choose to swim against the current, or control the flow of the river, you will exhaust yourself and drown. If you try to damn up the river, it will overflow the dam and destroy it. The river, the riptide, the Dao, cannot be stopped.

If, however, you choose to swim with the current you have choices as to which side you drift towards, whether you avoid rocks in the river, or low-hanging trees, or swim perpendicular to the riptide. You save your energy for the choices you make instead of wasting it on trying to control the flow of the river, or swimming against it.

Swimming against the river exhibits a Fear of Chaos, in an attempt to control the environment. It is an illusion, and it ain't gonna happen. Stop trying to control Chaos; turn around and let it be.

Chaos or Order?: a Matter of Perspective?

I was talking with a friend of mine at the farmers market the other week, on the topic of gardening. He admitted that he wasn't a particularly great gardner. I told him that the only thing I was really good at growing was weeds. He replied that he had always found the easiest way to eliminate weeds was through reclassification. Instead of calling them weeds, he just started calling them wildflowers.

BOOM! Problem solved!

My grandmother, Willie Bivans, had a similar mentality about weeds. One day, one of her neighbors looked over Willie's yard and commented in a particularly snarky tone, "Mrs. Bivans, your lawn is mostly weeds." Grandma was a tough girl raised in dirt floor shack in rural Georgia, so there was no way she was gonna let such an insult lie. She turned to look at her neighbor and said, in a biting tone, "It's *green* ain't it?" That was the end of the conversation.

This is a perfect illustration of how our mind creates the reality we experience. The difference between weeds and wildflowers, or weeds and *grass* is really a change in vocabulary. It is how we choose to see them. It has nothing to do with the reality of weeds versus wildflowers or grass. The plants are both things at the same time.

Our mind decides which reality we see. We can choose order or chaos depending on how you choose to see the world. There is a certain order within chaos itself. Look at the way nature unfolds around you, in cycles of seasons, birth and death. Look at the stars, planets, and galaxies in space. Is there no order to it? Of course there is. But there is chaos, as well.

I have a real Fear of Chaos. This is something I've only recently realized. I'm not sure how to get rid of it. I've made some progress on it, but I still have a long way to go. I think most people have it, and that it's a particularly human concern. It is a problem of reclassification.

The chaos we know becomes order, so is there really a difference? I don't think so. It's all in how we perceive it and the words we use to describe it. What is *new* is chaos, what is *old* is order. Chaos is just *change*. Change can be difficult, but it's necessary and inevitable.

It is through the crucible of chaos that all growth occurs. In order to grow, we have to accept that chaos is our friend, or at least accept that chaos is simply the way of things. The new chaos, or change will force us to grow. As we become accustomed to a change it becomes the new order. In turn, this leads us to become complacent, again, forcing us to again face new chaos to grow some more.

An acceptance of chaos is essential to human happiness and joy, to a peaceful life. We have an illusion that it is only through order that these things come into our lives. But that idea is a myth and a thief; it steals our joy and happiness and leaves us exhausted, like a swimmer swimming against a riptide. And there's only one end to that story: drowning.

Give up the struggle. Turn around and swim with the current and lose your Fear of Chaos. You might just make it to the beach.

MOVE THE SALT: SHRINKING THE CHANGE

As mentioned earlier in the book, one of the most difficult things about Process is that we become overwhelmed by all the details in achieving our goals, especially the big ones.

The best way to deal with large tasks is to break them down into smaller ones, even tiny ones. We need to *shrink* them down to get past the Fear of Starting.

Ask yourself, "What's the easiest thing I can do to break the inertia?"

So many times we get stuck because we're afraid of starting, mostly because we just don't know *where* to begin: what's the first step?

Just Move the Salt

"What the hell are you talking about?" you ask.

Yeah, I said, "Just move the salt."

Let me explain.

Have you ever had a kitchen sink and counter full of dirty dishes? Maybe the entire kitchen was a wreck after a party or a big second breakfast? Probably. I've certainly been in that situation.

The kitchen is such a mess that you don't even want to go in there and look at it, much less contemplate cleaning it up. I'm with ya. I feel that way nearly every day, though some days I don't have to clean it up—like this morning—because Patience beat me to it. It's nice when she does that, but I don't like to leave all the cleaning to her, since I'm a 21st Century man, and all.

How do I motivate myself to do something I don't really want to do?

I *trick* myself into doing it. I just move the salt. While I'm sitting in my big easy chair in my home office looking into the kitchen, moaning about the mess in there that I know I should attack, I stop and tell myself, "*Self, just go in there and put the salt away. Don't clean the kitchen, yet. Just put up the salt.*"

So, what happens? I go into the kitchen, turn on my little bluetooth, wireless speaker, walk into the living room and turn on some tunes. Then, I go back into the kitchen, look for the little, wooden salt cellar and I put it where it belongs.

That's it! Done!

Except that while putting up the salt, I see that the pepper is sitting nearby, so I put it away, too. Then the cereal box gets moved onto the kitchen table nearer to the pantry, and the tea pitcher magically makes its way into the fridge immediately followed by the bag full of bread, which miraculously ties itself back up and moves into its home position in the basket on the kitchen island.

Five minutes later, the entire kitchen is clean!

Why does this work? (And it definitely does.)

It works because I have just chosen to do something, anything, that will break the inertia of the Fear of Starting. All we have to do, in any situation, is to identify just one small thing in the process, the easiest, most doable, stress-free thing that we can do that is moving in the direction that we want to go.

For instance, let's say you're thinking of starting a new business. Let's say, to give it more concreteness, that's it's a pizza restaurant. Why pizza? Any example will do; ours is gonna be pizza. Deal with it.

So, you have a vision of what that pizza parlor will be, once it's up and running. It's gonna be awesome: none of that corner-cutting, chain-store-pizza crap! Hell no! Yours is gonna be an old-school, real ingredient, made to order, Pizza Palace! Great, you have the vision.

Now what?

That's where the problem comes in: the Fear of Starting. What do you do first?

If you can, make a list of all the things you *know* you have to accomplish before you're serving hot, fresh pizza to the neighborhood. Then, pick one of those things and do it. If you can't come up with that list, make of list of just one item:

1.   Right now, do a Google search on "How to open a pizza restaurant."

Then, complete the list! Go to your computer, or open up your Google search app on your phone or pad, and do it!

BOOM! You just moved the salt, my friend. Pretty soon you'll be the hottest pizza joint in town!

It's really that easy. Well, you still have to do all the other things on the list, but at least you've taken the first step, and that's a big step because it breaks the inertia.

The Fear of Starting can come back, however, at any point during the process. There are natural 'stopping points' in any process and it is important to try to avoid them, if possible.

Let's say you moved the salt; you Googled 'how to open a pizza restaurant' and a bunch of sites came up. You checked several of them out, read the content, saved them for later reference, or took really good notes, and now you have a better idea of what's involved in building a successful pizza joint.

Great. What's Next?

Did one of those sites lay out the steps in sequential order? Did they give you the next step in the process, i.e., 'where is the pepper shaker?' What is the pepper in the process? What's second, in other words? That's a natural stopping point, but don't be lulled into stopping. Grab another thing from the list and keep working.

Let's use another example: writing, since I know more about it than running a pizza joint.

One of the hardest things about writing is that you come to the end — of a chapter, an article, a book — and those are natural stopping points. So, most writers stop. But that's a bad practice to get into because then you have to break the inertia again, every time. You have to find, and move, the fuckin' salt every time you sit down to write.

I've experienced this many times. When I'm writing properly, I don't fall into that trap. I *do* fall into it, but only when I get complacent and lazy.

The way to avoid it when writing, is to set a certain time limit on when you write. Write like a madman or woman until the alarm goes off or the time you set appears on your clock. I don't always set an actual alarm, but I do write down the time I started and then usually write for one hour. When the alarm goes off, or the time is up, I stop writing.

I mean I *really* stop.

If I'm doing it correctly, I have to stop in the middle of a sentence. I don't even finish the idea I was working on at that moment, because the end of a sentence is, well, an END. It's a natural stopping point, ergo, not a place I should stop. If I just happen to be at the end of sentence when time runs out, fine, but I don't keep typing.

Now, I don't follow this rule with an iron fist or anything. I don't have an antique, writing Nazi — whatever the fuck that is — standing over me with a riding crop to lash my fingers if I don't stop typing in the middle of a sentence. So, sure, many times, I keep typing and finish the sentence. Sue me. Do as I say...forget what I actually do. Trust me, the best way to avoid writer's block, i.e., the Fear of Starting, is to never actually stop.

I read somewhere that a famous writer once said that when he finished the final draft of a book, he would take out another blank sheet of paper, put it in the typewriter and type the first sentence of the next book, and then be done for the day.

That's how momentum is gained and maintained. If you move the salt and then the pepper, pretty soon the entire kitchen will be clean, and you'll be serving up pepperonis and beer to happy pizza-eaters, or sending off your next best-seller!

While you're doing all that, stay focused on what you're doing NOW and stop worrying about what you're *not* doing.

YOU'RE NOT MISSING OUT

The Fear of Missing Out is a Catch22 Fear. We spend so much time rushing through life with the feeling that what we're doing right now isn't as important as what we *could* be doing. In reality, we miss out on our lives because we *fear* we're missing out on our lives. What a mess.

How to Banish this Fear?

The cure for the Fear of Missing Out is simple, if difficult to master:

1. **Acknowledge that you have it**. Take note when you start to worry about the other stuff on your To Do List.

2. **Meditate**: Put some attention on it. Perform a mini-meditation when it occurs. Think to yourself, "*Self, I'm drifting off into the future, and I'm afraid that what I'm doing isn't as important as what I* should *be doing.*" Then, as you notice that more often, reprogram your mind to focus on the present.

3. **Ask yourself some Afformation© questions**: "*Why am I enough? Why am I good enough! Why is what I'm doing right now*

the most important thing? Why is this the best place for me to be right now?"

This takes a lot of practice, but it is the best way to break the Fear of

Missing Out.

The more often you meditate, focusing on the present moment, on the Now, and the more you pose those positive questions to yourself, the faster the Fear of Missing Out will disappear.

Facing the Fear of Outcome: Into the Forest of the Future
"Courage is resistance to fear, mastery of fear—not the absence of fear."
—Mark Twain, author, master of biting wit, and #1 awesomeness
champion

Of all of the Branches of the Tree of Fear, the Fear of Outcome
seems to dominate our thoughts. We simply don't seem capable of
focusing our minds on the present. Instead, we constantly drift off
into the future. Planning for the future is fine, but worrying about it
is not. It serves no real purpose and will just screw up the present,
the only time we actually *have* in this life. As long as you have begun
the process of digging out your Fear of Inadequacy, the future will
seem less and less troublesome because you'll have the confidence
to face whatever comes.

But even the most confident person has days when they face
challenges looming in the future. Fear has a way of creeping back
into the mind, destroying our focus. Both Fear of Failure and Fear
of Success can hit us when we least expect it. For that reason, there
are a couple of things to keep in mind when that happens: courage
and vision.

BE THE KING OF THE FOREST: FACING FEAR WITH THE LION'S COURAGE

"If I were King of the Forest

not queen, not duke, not prince …" —Cowardly Lion in *The Wizard
of Oz*, movie, 1939

It was 12:35pm on Thursday.

Duke scanned the middle school lunchroom; his hands were

cold and sweaty.

Everyone was there. She was there. The time was now, or never.

If he hesitated, he'd never find the courage again, and all would be lost, even if this was a long shot from hell in the first place. So, he walked across the room and approached his target. Do or die, the time was now.

Five minutes earlier, Duke had secretly retrieved a bouquet of flowers from his locker. On the way to school that morning, I stopped at a convenience store so that Duke could purchase the flowers with his own money. Now, the time had come to deliver them, and ask the age-old, dreaded question.

Duke quickly crossed the distance from the stairs to the table where his intended sat. He tapped her on the shoulder, got down on a knee, and uttered the words he had run over and over in his mind all morning:

"Would you go out with me?"

Silence followed.

It seemed like the entire middle school was staring at him, and at her.

Five million years passed in dead silence.

Finally, she replied with the only thing that came to mind in that moment—faced with such a question from a friend who you just want to be friends with:

"What am I supposed to do with those?"

It wasn't the right thing to say, and the screaming sound of a diving fighter jet rang through the lunchroom with an echo, and the ripping, crumpling, crashing of metal meeting earth was pounding in Duke's ears and probably the ears of everyone around him.

Epic fail, and public as hell.

It was a waking nightmare.

Duke dropped the flowers and walked away, annihilated.

Meanwhile, in a classroom on the second floor, I was teaching a Latin class, knowing full well what was supposed to be going on downstairs. His mother was at work downtown, also worrying. I knew that the outcome was most likely to play out just as it did.

Duke had already posed the question to the girl a few days earlier, via text—not the recommended way—and had been told that she thought of him more as a brother. Ouch. How many of us have been on the receiving end of *that* response?

But Duke wasn't prepared to take *no* for an answer, not yet anyway. Not before giving it one more college try. So he did, and failed, miserably.

What really sucked, was that this was his first attempt to ask a girl out. He was an 8th grader, who had finally decided that girls are pretty okay, and not infested with cooties, or whatever they call it these days.

He had confided in me, a few days before the big Crash and Burn in the Lunchroom, about his 'text' attempt to ask her out. I told him that if she felt that way it was unlikely to change and that further attempts would probably be fruitless.

He was undeterred by the advice. Most people are.

The next day, he told me about his 'flowers at school' plan. I winced. I could see the whole thing play out in my mind, in vivid, flaming detail. But I did not try to stop him.

I'm old enough to know that you cannot offer unsolicited relationship advice and hope to have any real effect upon the other person's decision making process. Unless you agree with the decision they've already made, saying anything is a bad idea.

Why?

Because they aren't going to listen; you're not going to sway them to your point of view, and they're going to do it anyway.

Even if you *were* to sway them, what then?

What if Duke had *not* gone through with his plan? He certainly would not have gotten a date with the girl and he could have blamed me, forever, for his missed opportunity.

Second, if he had chosen to go ahead against the advice, he would have known—even though I might never have said it—that I was right, and could hit him at any moment with a dreaded, "*I told you so…*" which never does anyone any good.

So I remained silent, other than to ask a few questions, "*How do you plan to do this? Where? When?*" I didn't even want to tell Paysh, though I did, the day of. She was of a mind to step in and say something but I advised her that it would be a bad idea.

Somethings can only be learned in the wreckage of twisted metal and the searing flames of defeat.

What is the Lesson?

There's one more reason why I didn't step in to give him advice; crashing and burning at his age is a *good* thing. Everyone crashes and burns in life. In fact, we do it a lot, and that's okay. Remember 'fail fast'? It's a great way to learn, even if it hurts sometimes. That's why I allowed Duke to walk into that lunchroom in front of all of his peers, and fail.

What did he learn from this?

Tons. Some of it he won't fully realize for years, but he learned a few very important lessons from the experience right off the bat. One, that he has balls the size of Alaska. The courage it took to do what he did was an inspiration to me and Paysh and to everyone I've told the story to since.

I posted a short, audio version of the story on Anchor a day or two after the event. The response was viral. I think it ended up with over 100 responses. Friends and strangers chimed in to say that they were amazed and humbled by the courage that Duke displayed. Military combat veterans — men who had dodged bullets and bombs — praised him for his bravery. The ladies all wanted to know the 'end of the story.' Did he get the girl? What was the reaction of all the other girls and his friends?

For me, the biggest lesson was one about courage. I am still inspired by Duke's story. I told him that, while I had some pretty big balls and had done all kinds of courageous and brave things in my life, I would NEVER have done what he did. Hell no! To walk out in front of my entire middle school and ask a girl out with flowers? Not in a million years.

The fact that he did it is simply incredible. It is a lesson that he's never going to forget; I guarantee it. And if I had stepped in to stop it, it never would have happened. And it wasn't just me and my friends that recognized the courage it took; his *own* friends were texting him that evening to say things like,

"Dude! That was ballsy as hell!"

"I would never have done that! You're the man!"

Even the girl—who was his friend, after all—texted to say that she was sorry for hurting his feelings. While I think their friendship has been a bit awkward since then, they are not enemies. I've seen them talking and hanging out with their other friends together.

Another lesson that Duke learned (or will learn soon, I'm betting) is that his street value just went up with all the girls around that lunchroom table and the rest of the middle school.

How many girls dream of getting flowers from someone they like? Pretty much every one of them.

How many boys, or men for that matter, actually show up with them?

Not enough of us, that's for sure. I do, on occasion. (Which reminds me, I need to do it more often.) There were a lot of girls in that lunchroom watching what he did, probably thinking to themselves, "*Wow! Duke's a romantic! I wish my boyfriend would do that!*" My guess is that his act of bravery will pay off big in the future in the dating department. What do you think?

The lesson for the rest of us is that fearing is okay, even Fear is okay, or being afraid, but giving *in* to that Fear is not the way to go. Instead, let's suck up a little bit of Duke's courage and face those Fears. Let's kick them in the ass. It's okay if we fail. So what? We can always get back up and try something else the next day.

So, what's the rest of the story?

Well, when Duke got home that evening, he was depressed, devastated, and dejected. He was pissed off, mopey, and sullen.

That was to be expected.

But after supper, he was talking with Paysh in the kitchen about a field trip that the band was supposed to be going on the next day, during school hours. He didn't want to go, and she was hesitant to put pressure on him when he was so down. This is where I *did* step in, because I knew that letting him retreat into a shell would be a mistake.

"Duke!"

"What?" he answered in a depressed voice.

"Come in here."

He walked back into the office and I told him to sit down.

"Why don't you want to go on the field trip tomorrow?"

"I don't know; I just don't."

"Bullshit. That's not an answer. Why?" I knew why he didn't want to go, it was obvious, but I wanted him to say it out loud.

"I don't know, I just don't feel like it."

"Why? Because of what happened today?"

"Yeah, I guess so."

"Is the band going to be playing on this trip?"

"Yeah."

"Then you're going." I paused for a second before continuing. "You are an important part of that band. It's a team, and you cannot let down your teammates just because you're depressed and feel down right now. It isn't fair to them. More importantly, it won't help *you*. You're going on the trip."

"But.."

"But nothin'. You're gonna go, because it's your duty. It takes courage, but no more than going to class tomorrow would. You will feel better about the whole thing, if you go. You're just gonna have to trust me on this one. *I* know, and *you* don't, but you're gettin' ready to find out."

And he did find out.

He went, he had a great time and most of his depression, anger, and feelings of failure had subsided within 24 hours of the event.

Why?

Because he didn't sit still and roll around in his misery. He sucked up some courage, with a little kick in the ass from his parents and kept moving. It's the old, *"get back on the horse"* mentality. No Fear on Earth can withstand a tiny bit of courage. The second you suck up just a bit of courage, like Duke, like the Cowardly Lion, and turn to face your Fear, it blows away like so much smoke in the wind, or melts like the Wicked Witch of the West.

THE VISION OF OUR INNER HERO

As we discussed, the Fear of Failure isn't the only Outcome that can trip us up on our way to success. We can also have a Fear of Success itself.

If you encounter this Fear, or if you're already suffering from it and want to sweep it away, you have to visualize your inner hero, your higher self, and ask it some very important questions.

The following method comes from a good friend of mine on Anchor, Alida McDaniel, an intuitive life-coach. While researching to write this book, I posted an audio wave on Anchor about how to visualize success when you'd never really had it. Alida chimed in, thankfully, with a series of questions for me. During that process, we determined that I had a Fear of Success, along with a buffet of other Fears.

Alida challenged me to visualize my *Higher Self*, to imagine what life would be like once I reached my goals, as if I were a hero in my own story.

She posed five simple questions for me to answer and told me that, once I answered them, to start acting and *being* my higher self. That's the only way to attract success. We have to be in alignment with what we want or it won't come to us. Since I'm always up for a challenge, I sat down that afternoon and did just that.

When I began to answer the questions, I caught myself using the words, 'if' and 'would,' a lot. I stopped for a second, glanced over what I had written and realized that this was a projection of the very same Fear I was trying to overcome. So I went back and changed all those *ifs* and *woulds* into *whens* and *wills*!

Five Questions to Visualize Your Higher Self and Flog the Fear of Success:

Sit down with pen and paper and write, "*When I achieve my goals…*"

1.   **Who will I be? Will I be significantly different?**

2.   **What habits will I have?**

3.   **What thoughts will I have?**

4.   **What will be my story?**

5.   **What will be my work?**

Answer those questions and you'll be on your way to success.

Once you do all, or even a few, of the key steps in this book you're going to be on your way to the End of Fear Itself. If you need someone to help *guide* you through the Forest of Fear, don't forget there are lots of great coaches out there, like Alida, and me.

HIRING A PROFESSIONAL LUMBERJACK: THE VALUE OF A GREAT COACH

Sometimes, all the self-help books and 'best 5 steps' in the World don't seem to help us.

I've been there, for sure. Hell, that's part of the reason I began the journey to write this book: to walk through my own Forest of Fear. It's been a hell of a journey, for sure.

If you need a helping hand to get through your Fears, don't hesitate to reach out for help.

Hire a coach: a professional lumberjack.

A coach can help you with things, one on one, that are difficult or impossible to do on your own.

If you're lost in the Forest like Red Riding Hoood, you might need a trusty guide to get you to Grandma's house. Even more so to find and chop down your Tree of Fear. That's okay. We all need help sometimes. I sure do. If it were not for the help of a handful of awesome coaches, I wouldn't be here today writing this book and you wouldn't be reading it.

Without the assistance of Bobby Kountz, Greg Dickson, Alida McDaniel, Jamie Rautenberg, Luis Rivera, and my good friend, Justin Finkelstein, I would still be wandering around in the Forest listening to the baying of hungry wolves.

If you need help, hire someone. Beg, borrow, or liberate the funds to hire them. They're worth every damned penny. Some people spend thousands of dollars on self-help books, videos, and lots of other things that they think will make their life better, but never really invest in *themselves* by hiring a professional coach. If you're going to invest in something, what's more important than your own mental well-being?

If you really want to tackle Fear, hire ME. You can find me at www.stevebivans.com.

If you can't afford to hire a coach right now, try to find someone who'll do it for a trade-off, or for free. Maybe you *know* someone who's a coach and will help you out.

GOODIE BASKET FIVE: YOUR FEAR TREE REMOVAL KIT

- **Only YOU** have the power to End Fear Itself: your Fear.

- **Uncover your Fears** with the Shoveling Down Question: *"What do I need to be doing to achieve success in (fill in the blank) area of my life, right now, that I'm not currently doing?"*

- **Focus first** on your Fear of Inadequacy with positive *why* questions: *"Why am I so awesome?"*

- **Use your Axes** of Afformations©, Forgiveness, and Storytelling to chop up your other major Fears.

- **For your Fears of Loss:** Use the rakes of Mini-Meditations, Humor, and Gratitude to sweep them away.

- **For Fear of Process:** Remember to let go of Chaos, move the salt, and to stay in the Now.

- **For your Fears of Outcome:** Be the King of the Forest with courage, and make sure to visualize your inner Hero!

- **Hire a Lumberjack!:** If you still need help, make sure to invest in yourself and hire a professional coach to help you get through the Forest!

In a Forest of Fear: Just Keep Walkin'

"And remember, my sentimental friend, that a heart is not judged by how much you love, but by how much you are loved by others." —from the Wizard of Oz to the Tin Man, movie, 1939

Amber called me on Friday the 13th, 2015.
She was terrified.
"Dick is going to buy a gun." she said.
I could hear her voice tremble as she said it.
"You need to get the fuck out of there." I replied.
"I'm trying," she said, "I have a plan."
Amber did have a plan. With some encouragement from friends and family she finally left her husband.

But the wolves who live within the Forest of Fear don't easily give up on their prey. She needed a refuge, a place where he could not find her. For one night, the refuge was our home; Paysh and I took her in the next Friday, November 20th.

Along with her came stacks upon stacks of plastic storage bins jammed with colorful balloons.

Here was a woman trying to escape a deadly situation, surrounded by boxes of balloons in our living room. Why bring all of that? Because, despite her situation, she had a job to do. She was a performer, and Silly Miss Tilly had a purpose, to bring smiles and laughter to the world. That next day she had three birthday parties to attend.

I was flabbergasted! "Why don't you just call and cancel?" I asked. I mean here she was, trying to escape an abusive husband, and she was worrying about *work*!

But I missed something. The next day, I saw it, or maybe it's more accurate to say that I *experienced* it. Because to see it wasn't enough; it had to be felt. And what I saw and felt, I will never, ever forget.

Walking Through Hell

I leaned my throwing axe up against the center console and crawled into Amber's car.

It was about 8 o'clock in the morning, November 21st, 2015.

The car was parked in our garage to conceal it from the prying eyes of wandering wolves.

Amber crawled into the driver's seat, laughing at my iron companion, the Viking axe on the floorboard. "Oh my God!" she said, "Are you really going to bring that?"

"Abso-fuckin-lutely," I replied. "I don't take those kind of chances. It's not a gun, but I'm pretty good with it."

She laughed, turned the key and off we went down the road to her first gig which was about an hour out of town.

It was a long drive. She was an absolute emotional mess. She was shaking, crying and, in between all of that, second-guessing.

"My stomach is sinking," she would gasp, through sobs, "But I love him. Am I doing the right thing?"

"Yes," I assured her, over and over again, "You are. You just have to trust me on this one and keep going. On the other side of this hell is a world that is so awesome, so amazing, you can't even fathom it right now."

I'm not sure that any of my reassurances got through that day. But what *did* cut through the tears, the sinking feeling that her life was coming apart, was her life's mission: Smiles and Laughter.

When we finally found the first house, she parked the car next to the curb across the street from a large McMansion, and flipped a switch.

The Heart of the Tin Man: Power of Purpose

Something happened in the next couple of seconds that I cannot adequately explain. I can't put it into words but I witnessed it and experienced it, so I *know* it happened.

When she parked the car, she took a deep breath, got out, put on her gear, grabbed her stuff and headed for the door. Somewhere in that short walk, Amber the *wolf victim*, became Silly Miss Tilly the *children's performer*. It was like flipping a light switch. The transformation was instantaneous, and complete.

When she stepped into that first house, she was *on*. The fun returned, the smiles, the laughter, the happy children, the balloons. Everything was suddenly *right* in the world.

And she did that *three times* that day. In between each gig, she was an emotional wreck. But each time she stepped into the door of the house, her light came on. A light so bright that it was difficult to gaze into. At each stop, I went in with her to observe and be there in case something went wrong. But nothing went wrong in those spaces. She was in control. The wolf did not exist there.

It was the most inspiring thing I have ever seen. I am weeping as I write this in awe of that day. At all three houses, I had to excuse myself, more than once, to go into a bathroom to find some tissue or toilet paper to keep from weeping in front of everyone. They had *no idea* what Amber was going through that day. But I did. And I'll never forget her courage that day.

The beauty of Amber wasn't that she had no Fear. She had a truck-load of them: Fears to spare. No, her power came from her *heart*, and from a well-defined and internalized *purpose*, a mission statement: *Smiles and Laughter*. It is not just a catchy phrase on a business card or something she says with a fake smile to the kids. Amber *is* Smiles and Laughter. Her mission is *who she is*. It is the very heart of her identity. No matter how many doubts, Fears, or wolves come out of the woods, her purpose keeps her moving and the wolf can never touch that. In the face of the power of purpose, wolves turn and run, tails between legs.

A LIFE WITH PURPOSE: COURAGE OF THE LION, HEART OF THE TIN MAN

One thing a good life coach can do for you is to help you figure out your *Why*.

Do you know why you do what you do?

Do you have a life mission statement? or Life purpose?

Is it only a vague notion somewhere deep in your mind or have you actually written it out?

Amber's is written. It's on her website, on her business cards, and she can tell you in an instant if asked. Can you?

If the answer is *no*, then go to www.stevebivans.com, subscribe to my email list, and get your exclusive, free **Fear-Less Life Mission Worksheet**! You can do this at any time, of course. Just log in with your email address and I'll send you the password and link to the worksheet! Boom! Done!

With a Life Mission and No Fear, you'll be un-stopable.

Conclusion

A NEW FOREST

"All that is gold does not glitter,
Not all those who wander are lost;
The old that is strong does not wither,
Deep roots are not reached by the frost.
From the ashes a fire shall be woken,
A light from the shadows shall spring…" —J.R.R. Tolkien, *The Lord of*
the Rings

There is another seed.

Deep within the soul of the Forest, it sleeps.

It is a dream.

It lives in shadow.

It whispers in the night.

Wrapped in riddle,

It sings in songs.

Veiled in visions,

It rings in verse.

Preachers preach it. Dreamers dream it. Singers sing it.

Beneath the Forest floor there lies the seed that few ever find.
Long it lay dormant under frost, under roots, under the cursed Tree
of Fear, obscured by blackened seeds of our perceived
inadequacies.

It is the Seed of our Liberation.

The time has come to water that seed, to bring to life a *new*
Forest:

a Forest of *Freedom*.

A golden forest, glittering in the sun.

We will bend to Fear *no more*.

We are not weak.

We are strong beyond imagining.

We are beautiful.

We are children of light.

We are Smiles and Laughter.

Wolves flee before us.

fear *fears* Us.

We are fear-LESS.

We are Free.

Nothing can stand in the way of the Fearless. The world is ours, to transform, to rebuild, to renew. We will plant new trees, new forests. We shall shatter the chains of our past. The future shall run from us like mist in the wind. NOW is our time. NOW we will live in peace, in understanding, in acceptance, in compassion, in love, in freedom from fear.

Will you join me?

Will you walk with me?

Will you stand with me

upon this hill,

and do battle with fear?

Will you build a world of Freedom?

A new home?

Why?

Because, there's no place like home...

THANK YOU!

Thank you for reading this book!

I hope this book will help you to overcome your Fears and be all that you want to be.

If you enjoyed the book, do take a moment and leave a short review on Amazon! It really does help to keep the book at the top of the listings, and spread the word to more people. It's a small way that you can help to change the world.

And come visit me at www.stevebivans.com!

I write regular blog articles on many topics, including overcoming Fear. I'm also a FearLess Life Coach and Strategic Advisor. I work with both individuals and businesses to remove blocks to success.

If you enjoyed this book, check out my first book, ***Be a Hobbit, Save the Earth: the Guide to Sustainable Shire Living***. It's about how *you* can change the world, turn your neighborhood into a modern Shire, clean up the environment, and live happily ever after.

Don't forget to log in and claim your free Life Mission Worksheet at www.stevebivans.com!

Now that you're part of the Fear-Less World Movement, what better way to spread the word than with a kickass T-shirt! **Check out all the End of Fear Itself gear on Steve's website: www.stevebivans.com!**

ABOUT THE AUTHOR

Steve Bivans

is a FearLess Life Coach, Strategic Advisor, and Author of _Be a Hobbit, Save the Earth_, and _The End of Fear Itself_, both available on Amazon.

He has a master's degree in medieval history, is an expert on Viking Warfare and Culture, Tolkien's Middle Earth, the roasting and BBQing of meats, throwing kick-ass parties, and disrupting the _status quo_.

He is originally from the South Eastern U.S. (Florida and North Carolina), but now lives, happily, in Saint Paul, Minnesota with his girlfriend, Patience, her son Duke, Bubble the dog, and the Two Viking-Pirate Kitties: Punkin n Squish.

You can find Steve Bivans, all over the web, but his headquarters is at www.stevebivans.com

Made in the
USA
Monee, IL